Routledge Revivals

Health Care and Popular Medicine in Nineteenth Century England

Originally published in 1977, this book presents a selection of work by historians and sociologists on medicine and society in the 19th century. It concentrates on practitioners and patients, quackery and folk medicine, as elements in the social, cultural, political and economic structure of the community at large. The relevance of social history in medicine to the analysis of the role of medicine in society is discussed as well as the knowledge of sex and sexuality and the professionalisation of medicine.

Health Care and Popular Medicine in Nineteenth Century England

Essays in the Social History of Medicine

Edited by John Woodward and David Richards

Routledge
Taylor & Francis Group

First published in Great Britain in 1977 by Croom Helm Ltd.

This edition first published in 2025 by Routledge
4 Park Square, Milton Park, Abingdon, Oxon, OX14 4RN
and by Routledge
605 Third Avenue, New York, NY 10158.

Routledge is an imprint of the Taylor & Francis Group, an informa business

ISBN 13: 978-1-041-07903-3 (hbk)
ISBN 13: 978-1-003-64289-3 (ebk)
ISBN 13: 978-1-041-07934-7 (pbk)
Book DOI 10.4324/9781003642893

Health Care and Popular Medicine in Nineteenth Century England

ESSAYS IN THE SOCIAL HISTORY OF MEDICINE

Edited by JOHN WOODWARD
and DAVID RICHARDS

CROOM HELM LONDON

Croom Helm Ltd.
2-10 St John's Road, London SW11

ISBN 0-85664-321-1

Printed in Great Britain by Biddles Ltd, Guildford, Surrey

CONTENTS

TO CAROL AND TOM

CONTRIBUTORS

Janet Blackman is Lecturer in Economic and Social History at the University of Hull.

Ian Inkster is Lecturer in Economic History at the University of New South Wales.

Jean L'Esperance is a Librarian at the Department of Indian Affairs, Ottawa, Ontario.

Angus McLaren is Associate Professor of History at the University of Victoria, British Columbia.

David Richards is Head of the Department of Social Studies at Trent Polytechnic, Nottingham.

Ivan Waddington is Lecturer in Sociology at the University of Leicester.

Charles Webster is Reader in the History of Medicine, and Director of the Wellcome Unit for the History of Medicine at the University of Oxford.

John Woodward is Lecturer in Economic and Social History at the University of Sheffield.

PREFACE

The very success of historians of medicine in revealing, often with fine precision, the sources of modern scientific medicine, has tended to reduce their subject into a narrow specialisation capable of being appreciated only by an extremely limited audience. Thereby it has been too easy to lose sight of the potentially great historical importance of their subject matter. The recently formed Society for the Social History of Medicine seeks to redress this balance by promoting research into a wider spectrum of subjects relating to health, disease, medicine and public health. The Society depends for its success on drawing together workers from many different branches of medicine, history and the social sciences. The *Bulletin* of the Society already includes synopses of papers delivered at meetings.

In order to make current work in the field of the social history of medicine more fully available, John Woodward and David Richards have edited the present collection of papers, which are concerned with the interrelationships between medicine and society primarily in the first part of the nineteenth century. These papers concentrate on precisely the issues which tend to be neglected by the conventional history of medicine: medicine as it is related to the majority of practitioners and to the mass of the population. Nevertheless, it is such issues as the social role of the medical practitioner, intra-professional conflict, and attitudes towards sex and birth control, which were of the greatest contemporary relevance and which thereby contribute the most challenging and fruitful areas for historical investigation. The editors' introduction to this collection fully vindicates the work of the Society and it is hoped that this volume will be the prelude to further publications of this kind.

Charles Webster

'It is our duty to remember at all times and anew that medicine is not only a science, but also the art of letting our own individuality interact with the individuality of the patient.'

Albert Schweitzer

'There are only two classes of mankind in the world - doctors and patients.'

Rudyard Kipling —'A Doctor's Work'

'There are no diseases, there are only patients.'

Salvador De Madariaga Y Rojo
Essays with a Purpose - 'On Medicine'

'The medical profession is unconsciously irritated by lay knowledge.'

John Steinbeck - East of Eden

'That society which can reduce professional intervention to the minimum will provide for the best conditions of health.'

Ivan Illich - Medical Nemesis

INTRODUCTION

Health, and health services have in recent years become areas of major social and economic concern in both industrialised and developing countries. This has prompted comparative analyses, over both time and place, of the manner in which health has been perceived, and in which health services have been developed, delivered and woven into the everyday social fabric. Less evident, however, has been any co-ordinated effort at detailing the social processes and pressures which underpin these perceptions and developments. Health care facilities, like social welfare provision, have evolved in response to a complex battery of needs, demands and social, economic and political pressures. Remarkably little work in the history of medicine has, however, focused in any depth upon the precise social processes which have encouraged or hindered the application of medical science in the community.

This collection of essays attempts a positive realignment towards a greater emphasis on the social aspects of health, and medical care. In presenting a selection of current work, by both historians and sociologists, on the British experience in the nineteenth century, this volume seeks to delineate and encourage a social history of medicine. Although the perspectives presented deal predominantly with one country over one particular century, it is to be hoped that the approaches outlined in this book will be symptomatic of a burgeoning interest in the area, not only in Britain but also in North America, Europe and elsewhere. As the editors indicate in their opening essay, there have already been some seminal studies in North America by Sigerist, Rosen and others, who have urged a social history of medicine. The development of such an approach has been strangely neglected in Britain. Nonetheless, from a reading of the literature emanating from a wide range of disciplines and countries, it is clear that there are many points of departure from which historians and social scientists may contribute to our chosen field. A knowledge and awareness of the social history of medicine, and of allied health sciences and services, will contribute to a greater understanding of the dynamic nature of societies and cultures, and of the changing roles of patients, medical practitioners and systems of health care.

There are thus many themes to the social history of medicine: in order to introduce this comparatively new area of study, it has, however, been felt advantageous in this book to select after some deliberation two particular themes – knowledge of sex and sexuality, and professionalisation in medicine. It is evident that each of the selected themes is capable of differing interpretations, uses and analyses. The essays themselves should be seen as statements of present and continuing interest rather than as final and complete expositions. The aim, therefore, is for them to serve not only as catalysts for future research and studies in the contributing disciplines but also as initial explanations and interpretations of the role of medicine in society.

The editors, in their opening essay, attempt to develop these preliminary remarks, define more precisely the social history of medicine, and indicate a number of fruitful areas for research. The essay reflects their own backgrounds, showing both historical and sociological frameworks and interpretations, and seeks to synthesise many of the themes, contained within the existing literature, which might be considered of especial relevance to medicine in society. This can only be an initial exploration of what is clearly a vast and expanding subject, involving a cognisance of many apparently disparate but nevertheless interrelated disciplines and perspectives. In short it is the editors' intention to open up a potentially fertile field where only a few seeds have been sown, and where indeed some, through a lack of cross-fertilisation, have failed to germinate. It is, however, to be hoped that the essays from the other contributors to the volume show that a fruitful cross-fertilisation of disciplines is not only possible but also beneficial.

There then follow two essays, by Janet Blackman and by Angus McLaren, devoted to the theme of knowledge of sex and sexuality. These subjects, though intrinsically interesting in their own right, have however, very much more to offer the social historian of medicine. Both essays indicate not only the basic facts about knowledge of birth control and pregnancy, but also act as barometers of ideas on sexual relations and childbirth. Blackman, by studying the various editions of a popular lay manual – *Aristotle's Works* – describes the way in which scientific ideas and information were absorbed into popular culture. As scientific knowledge regarding procreation and pregnancy developed, such information was differentially distilled, transmitted and perceived. The medical profession in the nineteenth century – and indeed in the early twentieth – was loath to accept the utility of such a manual for the lay public and, moreover, preferred to preserve an aura of mystery about pregnancy and childbirth. This is an important lesson to be learnt even today in the field of health education, for it is clear that knowledge in itself can be an insufficient stimulant to action by the general public. As Blackman herself concludes, her concern is 'with collective behaviour, and with widespread attitudes towards and general understanding of knowledge provided by the professional and the privileged elite, and how the working-class came to absorb or reject such information in their own lives'. McLaren uses birth control in the early years of the nineteenth century to illustrate a patient-initiated approach. He demonstrates the public's ignorance of and demand for instruction in sexual matters, particularly birth control. The medical profession was refusing to recognise birth control as a medical question with which it should involve itself, thereby leaving the area free for the use of popular literature, quack treatments and recommendations. Popular manuals and quackery satisfied the rising demand for knowledge, especially among the lower classes, who were not gaining access to the medical establishment. There thus arose what McLaren has described as a self-help medical movement, which 'was to instil in the layman a faith in himself and his ability to control his own life'. There were, evidently, two contrasting groups within society both seeking to conquer disease — doctors believing in reforming their profession, and lay individuals in reforming society.

Jean L'Esperance, in her synthesis of contemporary views regarding female sexuality and the role of women in society, emphasises the growing desire for knowledge, which has been clearly demonstrated in the previous two papers. Within the context of the Victorian 'double standard' of sexual morality, she shows that women were becoming increasingly aware of their own sexuality, and describes how this led to a growing assertion for a more positive role in society. She takes as her examples the campaigns to gain recognition for women as doctors, nurses and midwives. Her essay draws attention to the need 'to understand changes in beliefs regarding sexuality in the context of a relationship between the professionalisation process and the changing structure of sexual division in society'. Thus the new role of women may be seen as 'marginal' — a concept developed in a parallel context in the following paper. This essay on women and doctors admirably bridges the twin themes considered in this collection — namely knowledge of sex and sexuality, and professionalisation in medicine.

The final two essays in this symposium develop the theme of professionalisation within medicine in the first half of the nineteenth century. Ian Inkster describes aspects of the social role of the medical community — using, in a historical setting, the example of Sheffield for a micro-analysis of the concept of 'marginality'. He demonstrates that a professionalising group was wholly aware of its sensitive social position and also analyses the relationship of provincial medical men to the local community, economy and society. It is clear that there existed in Sheffield a 'social network', or scientific community, whose members, consisting particularly of medical practitioners, were involved in the establishment and management of many of the social, educational, medical and scientific institutions in the area. A partial verification of his contention is provided by his brief examination of such phenomena in another provincial town, Derby. This involvement of medical men in the community is shown to be a mechanism which facilitated professional recognition in the wider society and marked a further step in the acceptance of medicine as a truly professional occupation. The professionalisation process, described by Inkster, is taken up in a wider context by Ivan Waddington, whose essay is primarily concerned with changing relationships within the medical community itself, and in particular with that between consultants and general practitioners. Although it has been commonly considered that the medical profession in the first half of the nineteenth century was rigidly structured into three categories, namely physicians, surgeons and apothecaries, Waddington introduces a new facet for any analysis of this group. By considering the careers and modes of practice of several prominent medical men, he draws attention to the development of the role of 'general practitioners', and the concomitant intra-professional conflicts with 'consultants'. As he concludes, 'it is only by analysing the socially structured tensions within a profession that we can understand why and how the institutional framework emerged and changed from period to period'.

The editors' aim in bringing together these essays has been to indicate, and to offer some examples of, a new approach to the understanding of past society by using the concept of what can be termed ' a social history of medicine'. It is evident that many 'traditional' studies in the history of medicine and medical science, and of the medical profession have failed to take sufficient account of the parts played by both practitioners and patients as elements in the social, cultural, political and economic structure of the community at large. Furthermore, and since it is clear that there were many who did not even progress to 'patienthood', there has been a significant lack of focus on lay individuals, their perceptions of illness, disease and doctors, their resort to quack and folk medicine, and their use of popular literature and remedies. As the opening essay explains, there is an important need for historical studies which view medicine, not merely from a medical or professional perspective, but from that of the typical contemporary man or woman. How did health and disease and health- or sickness-related behaviour fit in with the everyday pattern of life? By revealing a wider understanding of this area, and by demonstrating the way in which the practice of medicine, medical knowledge and experimentation, scientific enquiry, and the provision of health care facilities have advanced in relation to other aspects of society, a social history of medicine can provide important historical and social scientific data. An understanding of the impact of changes in these areas, together with that of social ideas and values, on physical and mental conditions of well-being and health, will facilitate an enhanced explanation of both times past and present, and hopefully lead to improvement in and development of health care in the future.

At this point in an introductory essay it is customary to make a number of acknowledgements – we are only too pleased to follow in this tradition. Indeed the impetus for both this volume and the new approach to the history of medicine has come from discussions, both formal and informal, with many friends and colleagues (representing a wide range of disciplines) in Britain and elsewhere. We are very conscious of the debt we owe to fellow members of the Society for the Social History of Medicine – in particular its founders, Ruth Hodgkinson, Huw Francis and Sidney Chave, and its current President – Charles Webster. The implementation of our ideas would not have been possible without the co-operation of our contributors whose concepts and views have helped to mould our own thoughts. We also wish to acknowledge the additional assistance given by Ivan Waddington and Janet Blackman in reviewing manuscripts and helping to focus our attention on the selected themes. We also owe a special debt to George Rosen, whose many scholarly publications have done so much to enhance the development of socio-historical studies in the field of health, and have, in particular, stimulated us to assemble this collection of essays. The writing of our own essay, and the checking of references has greatly benefited from our access to the university libraries at Sheffield and Nottingham, and to the library at the Wellcome Institute for the History of Medicine, London, where Eric Freeman, Robin Price and Gordon Wilson have revived our spirits with appropriate fuel, and generally encouraged us in our task. We also realise that this book would not have been completed without assistance from British Rail, whose frequent delays and engine-failures on the St Pancras-Nottingham-Sheffield line provided us with more than ample opportunity for reflection, discussion and elaboration of our ideas. Indeed the behaviour of the hordes of exuberant and effusive Scotsmen, who boarded the overnight train to Glasgow at Kettering, very nearly convinced us to add in to our collection a paper on the social history of alcoholism. This, however, we leave for another malt.

Last but not least special thanks must be given to Carol Richards, not only for her accurate and speedy typing of our untidy and often illegible manuscripts, but also for providing meals on demand for us at unsociable hours. The start of her tennis season finally persuaded us that we ought to finish this book.

John Woodward, *University of Sheffield*

David Richards, *Trent Polytechnic*

April 1976.

1 TOWARDS A SOCIAL HISTORY OF MEDICINE

John Woodward and David Richards

This essay attempts to define, delineate and develop what has been a largely neglected area of co-operation between history, medicine and the social sciences. In urging a synthesis of historical and sociological perspectives to medicine, this paper has the ambitious aim of re-orientating a social history of medicine. It uses medicine, and its allied health sciences, as a theme for the elaboration of historical and sociological knowledge, and in so doing, endeavours to encourage a wider historical understanding of the interrelationships between man, medicine and society. A sympathetic liaison between history and sociology has been urged by many writers, of whom perhaps E.H.Carr has expressed it most poignantly: '. . . the more sociological history becomes, and the more historical sociology becomes, the better for both'.[1] In essence the need has been to develop a fusion between studies of different phenomena at one point in time, and of the same phenomenon over different periods. The social history of medicine will seek to incorporate these two elements of study in developing a deeper analysis of the role of medicine in society. One further preliminary comment is necessary: sadly, the social history of medicine has often been equated with the history of social medicine. This latter specialism, although involving a penetrating examination of epidemiology and the distribution of disease in society, forms but a part of the social history of medicine, which concerns itself with more far-reaching interrelationships between medicine and society and not merely, as does the latter, with the field of public health and preventive medicine. Or as George Rosen put it in his Presidential Address to the Society for the Social History of Medicine:

> The social history of health and disease is therefore more than a study of medical problems. . . . It requires as well an understanding of the factors – economic conditions, occupation, income, housing, nutrition, family structure and others – which create or influence health problems, and of the ways in which they operate.[2]

The first section of the essay is devoted to a brief statement concerning the lack of social emphasis of much work in the history of medicine. The following two sections describe some of the fields of interest and commitment of the historian and sociologist and outline individual studies in these disciplines which have, albeit sometimes unconsciously, contributed to the development of both a social history of medicine, and a historical sociology of medicine. The concluding section attempts to draw together various threads from the medical, historical and sociological literature and to point to some areas for future joint research endeavour. A deeper, more committed and analytical social history of medicine will permit a wider understanding of medicine, history and society. Adoption of any but an interdisciplinary perspective will be to miss many of the subtleties of the situation. This is not, however, to suggest that doctors, historians and sociologists should be any less committed to their own specialisms, but rather that a total explanation of the development of medicine in society will be dependent on a realisation of the importance of the interrelationships between the three disciplines. In Britain, at least, at the present time many studies in the field have lacked evidence of such a multi-sided approach, and of a wide and critical reading of the parallel literature. Such a symbiosis would seem by contrast, to be more apparent in North America, as the writings of Sigerist, Rosen, Shryock, Pellegrino and others amply demonstrate. It is to be hoped then that this essay will underline the full meaning suggested by George Rosen in his review of Henry Sigerist's *A History of Medicine:* '. . . medicine is an activity whose development can be most fully understood only when considered in relation to the network of social interaction within which it occurs'.[3]

The history of medicine has a long and distinguished pedigree, and yet its status and influence on areas both outside, and indeed also inside medicine has been of limited consequence. Much of the approach of the history of medicine has been based, until recently, on a mere collection of facts which have been displayed either chronologically or thematically. Such a tendency is clearly shown in the works of, say, Garrison, Osler, Cumston, Singer, Guthrie, Castiglioni and Pazzini.[4] In the words of one critic:

> Medical theory, literature and practice occupy focal points in the presentation; less attention is paid to the history of the medical profession and still less to the history of community health. While the significance of social factors and conditions are recognised, this aspect is relegated to the very periphery of the picture.[5]

This comment on the traditional iatrocentric approach to the history of medicine is really the starting point of this discussion. The history of medicine has been 'doctor' orientated. It has been studied by doctors for doctors, and has been primarily about doctors. If it has not been about doctors, it has been about the history of science as it impinges upon medicine. Science, however, as Sigerist noted, can only be 'one aspect of medicine and there can be a great many aspects the history of which has to be investigated'.[6] Even when dealing with the personalities of medicine, the biographies tend to study only the famous – nonetheless the bulk of medicine was and is carried out by individuals who do not have national or international reputations. It is clear that, notwithstanding a sense of academic scholarship, the history of medicine has been seen in extremely narrow terms. Histories of technical achievement, of medical institutions, of progress of treatment against disease, and of the medical and allied professions, almost without exception, are self-contained within medicine – they neither look at the patient and the community nor at the areas outside medicine upon which their work impinges – e.g. legislation (medical or non-medical) or changes in status groups in society. In short, much of the history of medicine has focused on medical discoveries and personalities, and provided little information on social organisation or the reasons for developments and discoveries. One event does not lead inexorably on to the next – as many studies would suggest. This is not to state that histories of medicine and of science are not without value, but merely to underline the complementary nature of studying, inter alia, the application and interpretation of progress in these areas in the wider society.

Some thirty years ago one perceptive historian – Charles Mullett – suggested that the historian of medicine needed to enjoy a healthy scepticism about his subject and to remember that 'disease, its threat, mortality and general consequences, has influenced the course of history far more than matters often receiving greater and more serious attention'.[7] He believed that there were a number of areas which needed particular attention:

(a) studies of pandemics 'that had certain persistent elements, that had revolutionary effects on society in all its forms, that recurred year after year. These studies will supply comparative data and integrate medicine and civilisation'.[8]

(b) studies of 'diseases that survived through the ages arousing the antidotal concern of physicians and governments'.[9]

(c) studies of acute or occupational diseases, and studies of diseases not conspicuously fatal 'but wearing down health and morale, costing money, and complicating social, economic and political problems'.[10]

(d) studies of the relationship between the environment, including climate, and disease, and

(e) studies in comparative pathology.

This emphasis on disease has great possibilities for it gets outside the narrow field of clinical medicine as practised by doctors, but very few historians have really explored the social connotations of disease. The plague and cholera are two great endemic diseases, which have been examined,[11] and Rosen has made a classic study of one of the occupational diseases, miners' disease.[12] In his introduction to this latter study Sigerist wrote that

> . . . the history of occupational diseases is infinitely more than medical history. Of course the more medicine knew about the causes and nature of such disease, the more effectively they could be prevented. But hazards and diseases change with developing industries and whether any use was made of medical knowledge did not depend so much on the physicians as on the social organisation under which the labourer performed his task. The history of occupational diseases, therefore, reflects as in a mirror the history of industry and the history of labour, in other words some of the most important chapters in the history of human civilisation. It not only illustrates most dramatically the development of the Industrial Revolution but also the accompanying medical and social reforms gained by the labouring class.[13]

It is the wider social context which is of major significance – a point which is stressed constantly in this essay.

Historians of medicine have produced many biographies – and autobiographies – of medical men. It is clear, however, that very few who practise medicine are famous – a relative term which is often applied for other than medical reasons. Again this is not to suggest that such studies are not without interest or value, but rather to make the point that they may not necessarily convey an exact impression of what constituted the work of the typical medical man at any particular age. These biographies are usually chronological accounts which barely look beyond the subject's social grouping. Nonetheless they may indeed provide information for an examination of professionalisation, and of the progress of health legislation – in other words they may serve as sources of data for wider socio-historical analysis. In themselves, however, many of the biographies make but little reference to the social context in which their subjects practised medicine.

Again there have been many histories of public health, and of social and preventive medicine. This is an area which can be treated on many levels. Much of the literature in this area is written as straight administrational and legislative history. This can be seen at the national level, as in William Ashworth's *The Genesis of Modern British Town Planning,* or at local level in Asa Briggs' *History of Birmingham.*[14] If it is not legislation, it is 'sewers and drains' with a technical history about hydraulics and plumbing included. Significantly the kind of public health history which has emerged in recent years, and yet not been written by doctors, has opened up the whole area. Indicative of this development have been the biographies of Edwin Chadwick by Lewis and Finer, and of Sir John Simon by Royston Lambert.[15] In these perceptive books the implications of the lives and work of these key figures are studied. It is clear that analyses of this standard are of prime importance, not only for the social history of medicine, but also for the development of social administration. Again this is to stress the importance of the confluence of interests, and of the gains to be made from a cross-fertilisation of disciplines.

It is not the purpose of this essay to attempt a wider critique of the field of the history of medicine, other than to draw attention to the lack of attention and appreciation of the social context. Social history has, it is clear, not been without its critics – nonetheless it has moved a long way from the pioneering studies by Trevelyan. The concern is no longer merely with the collection and assembly of facts but with their interpretation. Furthermore and significantly the facts have been collected by members of other disciplines, for it would be absurd to suggest that all facts from the past can only be studied by the trained historian. Thus E.J. Hobsbawm, in an essay on social history, quotes Fustel de Coulanges: '. . . history is not the accumulation of events of all kinds which occurred in the past. It is the science of human societies.'[16] Hobsbawm continues:

> We are concerned not only with structures and their mechanisms of persistence and change, and with the general possibilities and patterns of their transformations, but also with what actually happened . . . It is the history of societies as well as of human society . . . or of certain types of society and their possible relationships . . . or of the general development of humanity considered as a whole.[17]

There has been considerable discussion, along these lines, about the nature of history, and the specialism termed social history. Is there, however, any distinction between the two? When E.H. Carr produced his incisive *What is History?* in 1961, he wrote as follows: 'To enable man to understand the society of the past and to increase his mastery over the society of the present is the dual function of history.'[18] This emphasis on the use of history in its social context pervades many of the discussions and the work of Harold Perkin and Asa Briggs.[19] If a definition of history is attempted, there are perhaps three important contexts which must be understood:

> History is, first of all, the custodian of the collective memory, and as such performs the important function of nourishing the collective ego. Second, it is in all societies a primary vehicle of the socialisation of the young, teaching them the past so that they may know who they are, and behave appropriately in the present. Third, it is the branch of inquiry that seeks to arrive at an accurate account and valid understanding of the past.[20]

This statement appears to put a massive responsibility on the historian. How is he to undertake his task? Some historians, particularly those of a Marxist persuasion, argue that 'the history of society cannot be written by applying the meagre available models from other sciences: it requires the construction of adequate new ones – or at least. . . the development of existing sketches into models'.[21] Is this really being fair to others who have developed models of society? There are many sociologists who have developed their own models, which may prove useful in an examination of society. Perhaps the two who have really looked at the past in Britain in a new way are Neil Smelser, in his study of textile workers during the Industrial Revolution, and Michael Anderson, in his study of family structure in nineteenth-century Preston.[22] There have, in addition, been the many studies derived from Weber and Tawney on the development of entrepreneurship, culminating in the 1960s with the work of McClelland and Hagen.[23] The historian should not be too proud but should be prepared to make use of the skills and models available in other sciences. Again the lesson for the social historian of medicine seems clear.

As history has developed its own identity it has also created within its new specialisms and areas of interest. Provided that the limitations of historical research are recognised, these specialisms can be of paramount value in determining the past and understanding the present. The facts of history never occur in a pure form – or as Carr has put it: 'Study the historian before you begin to study the facts.'[24] There is thus an important need for a critical understanding, albeit through the eyes of the present, of not only the interpreter of facts, but also of the so-called facts themselves. Many studies in the field under review have seemingly been blind to such biases.

Asa Briggs has suggested six areas for specialist development by the social historian.[25] Although, in his own essay, he was concerned with the history of education, the social history of medicine would equally fit into his six categories: (1) local history, (2) comparative history, (3) quantitative history, (4) 'new' social history, (5) political history, and (6) intellectual and cultural history. In an effort to stimulate further development of a social history of medicine a selective review of pertinent historical studies in each of these areas will follow. The aim is not to provide a complete catalogue of research but rather to act as a catalyst for future study, and to draw attention to focal points and approaches.

To consider Briggs' first area: the study of local history has in recent times become more professional and less antiquarian. The antiquarian approach of describing institutions and personalities, however, is of some value to the historian, in establishing the facts. Armed with these facts the historian can progress to examining processes and structures, and discovering the continuities and discontinuities over time. Instead of generalising from national legislation and society, the work of the local historian can illustrate and illuminate more fully the life of the people. National history, after all, draws on a collection of local histories. Within the field of medicine it is possible to study the impact of national legislation, often permissive, on the local community, and also to see the pressure from local level towards the centre. One of the topics in which this is particularly clear is that of the impact of both endemic and epidemic disease. A pioneering effort is that of Bertrand on the outbreak of plague in Marseilles in 1720.[26] This is an account of an outbreak in which 60,000 out of 90,000 people contracted the disease, and where only 10,000 recovered. In Biraben's view:

> The extent of this extraordinary death toll in a rapidly developing town brought about in a matter of weeks first of all economic then administrative disorganisation and finally such social disintegration that it would be difficult to find many comparable cases in modern times.[27]

Bertrand, as a physician, 'wished to maintain his position, sharing with his contemporaries those conceits of class or profession which he thought to place him above the common sort'.[28] This is a fascinating study not just for the account of the epidemic itself, but for its insight into social relationships and perceptions of disease. Bertrand relates how the municipal authorities tried, principally for commercial reasons, to understate the severity and the nature of the outbreak:

> Believing strongly with the people and many doctors, that fear is the main agent in the spread of disease, they attacked the town's qualified doctors, spreading the rumour that the latter intended to terrorise the population in order to aggravate contagion and increase their earnings.[29]

Biraben concludes his introduction by describing Bertrand's work as, 'a sociological document which the emphatic writings of the period on the plague in Marseilles rarely equal, and which greatly reinforces its historical or medical interest'.[30]

In many ways the examination of this one study draws out the other approaches to history, which Briggs has noted. As there may be similarities and differences in response between urban and rural communities, and between regions within one country, there may also be the same comparisons to be made over national boundaries. The structures and processes of history can be strongly highlighted by the comparative method: 'When an analyst cannot experiment with his subject matter through replication, establishment of controls, and the manipulation of variables, then he resorts to the comparative method in the hope of achieving the same explanatory.'[31] An excellent example of the use of the comparative method can be seen in Post's recent study of disease and famine in Europe.[32] In making a survey of the outbreak of bubonic plague in Europe after the Napoleonic Wars, Post comments that

> . . . unlike the history of typhus, the evidence on plague fails to support the view of increasing natural immunity among European populations. Neither does the historical record confirm the supposed linkage of plague and malnutrition. Those historians who have advanced a case for autonomous plague epidemics are probably justified in this position. The limited knowledge now available indicates an antagonistic rather than a synergistic relationship between protein deficiency and resistance to infection from the plague bacillus.[33]

Although this is a specific example, related to one disease, further comparative studies are made for other diseases, and over other territories, and there is an important conclusion for the historian:

> The evidence suggests that any model of explanation covering famine, mortality and epidemic disease cannot be reduced to the simple interaction between nutrition and infection. It is equally clear that in the case of an autonomous zootic disease like plague, or a communicable human disease like typhus, inevitably social, economic and political conditions as well as biological and meteorological parameters are involved. Neither is escape from bubonic plague or epidemic typhus quite as automatic as the French plague commission believed, when it concluded that'the progress of civilisation' and the application of the rules of hygiene would prevent epidemics. The economically developed United Kingdom and Switzerland as well as backward Italy failed to control severe typhus epidemics. Yet Britain and Switzerland were as modernised as France and the Netherlands, and more so than Austria and many German states. Switzerland failed to minimise the rise in mortality because political decentralisation reduced the resources that could potentially have been allocated to those cantons disproportionately weighed down by the subsistence crisis and because decentralisation led to administrative competition instead of co-operation. The United Kingdom failed to control famine and epidemic disease in Ireland essentially because *laissez-faire* and individualistic guidelines created an administrative blind-spot. The same administrative premises permitted both the typhus epidemic and social distress to assume major proportions in England, Scotland and Wales. However in Britain, unlike Ireland and Italy, economic development produced a modicum of relief, and together with the sanitary barriers ensuing from the process of modernisation prevented a devastating increase in the death rate.[34]

The virtue of this quotation is that it, yet again, brings together a number of the approaches proposed by Briggs, and introduces some themes which will be discussed in later sections of this essay.

Quantitative history, sometimes called 'quanto-history', is necessary for any understanding of the past, not just for the stastics but to know what has to be analysed. The specialism most closely related to medicine is that of historical demography.[35] Demography has developed as a historical science from the early collections of pre-census parochial data, and the subsequent reworking of the parish register abstracts. In attempting to assess the contribution of medicine and of changes in the impact of disease to population growth in Britain from the middle of the eighteenth century, there has been much controversy. Buer and Talbot Griffith in the 1920s suggested that the growth of hospitals and medical care in the eighteenth century contributed to a fall in mortality.[36] This idea was not to be seriously challenged until the 1950s, when McKeown and Brown disputed the favourable impact of medicine and substituted a far more pessimistic viewpoint.[37] Two aspects of this influential paper have recently come under greater scrutiny. Inoculation, rather than vaccination, against smallpox in the eighteenth century has been suggested as a major factor in promoting a reduction in mortality, and the 'detrimental' role of hospitals has been seriously questioned by examining the statistical evidence of the hospitals themselves.[38] As yet the debate has not been conclusively finalised and it is evident that further and deeper research, particularly from a range of local sources in order to offer a comparative judgement, has to be undertaken. Other aspects of demography in relation to disease have been undertaken, using parish registers, by for example D.E.C. Eversley and J.D. Chambers.[39] These studies have indicated how local variations in the incidence and impact of epidemic disease had important regional consequences. Although all these papers contain much statistical material, in recent years there has been a complete reappraisal and reworking of parochial data. The work of the Cambridge Group for the History of Population and Social Structure, following the lead given in France, has enabled close study to be made of the structure of families, class divisions, and the incidence of disease and famine.[40]

An entirely different approach to statistics can be seen in analysing the nineteenth-century predilection for the collection of such material for social and moral purposes. By examining the growth of the 'statistical movement' from the 1830s, M.J. Cullen has sought to demonstrate that there was a distinguishing philosophy among such men as William Farr, William Guy, and later Charles Booth.[41] The concern with sanitary statistics and other such material leads Cullen to the conclusion that: 'The widespread but short-lived concern with improvement by numbers was a significant movement of the period: its permanent legacy was not so much a new moral order as the indigenous tradition of empirical social research characteristic of British sociology.'[42] Thus the study of such a movement indicates yet another field of interest to which this essay will return, namely intellectual history.

The importance of quantitative social history has been stressed by

S.P. Hays who has noted trends in a movement towards historical social research, involving (a) new concepts, which consider not single happenings but events as part of a social process, (b) a distinctive method which is systematic rather than intuitive, and (c) the use of new techniques such as statistics and computer analyses.[43] Interaction between the social sciences and history, using quantitative methods, has 'far more to offer than the substitution of an overload of quantitative data for an overload of qualitative date. It provides opportunities for conceptual reconstruction and for theory development through comparative method'.[44]

Social history itself has been growing in stature by the use of concepts derived from sociology, psychology and anthropology. Much of the new work has concentrated on discerning the attitudes and feelings of the mass of the people – 'history from below'.[45] There has been little investigation, however, of the perceptions of the ordinary man or woman regarding health, disease and medical care. Further discussion of this area follows in a later section of this paper which considers the development of a historical sociology of medicine. One particular area which has come to prominence is that of 'psychohistory'.[46] Attempts have been made to decipher and understand the personalities, emotions and mental aptitudes of prominent people and their children. D.R. Allen has, for example, applied some of the concepts of psychoanalytical psychology to understanding data from a number of biographical studies of Florence Nightingale. The main theme of his study is that she achieved greatness through her efforts to control the basic conflicts of her personality.[47] The focus of psychohistory on biographical analysis, together with a deeper study of group and 'movement' behaviour, will permit a wider interpretation of many key figures in the development of health professions and services.

'Traditional' political history has concentrated on dates, individuals and legislation without seeing such activities in a wider context, particularly the accretion of administrative processes, the nature of decision-making and the role of organisation. In this context the growth of legislation, and its nature, in the field of public health have important relevance. Studies of the growing awareness of public health problems in nineteenth-century Britain have moved away from mere descriptions of squalor and disease, and 'sewers and drains', towards more thorough-going analyses of the pressures at central and local level for and against legislation. These discussions make an important contribution to the continuing debate over *laissez-faire* versus state intervention – a debate sparked off by Oliver MacDonagh's seminal paper reappraising the

'Nineteenth Century Revolution in Government'.[48] Much comment has followed: in the field of health Novak has proposed an alternative approach.[49]

In the public health field it has become increasingly clear that only an incremental approach could be made:

> Local initiative and central administrative growth created the patchwork, *ad hoc,* pragmatic, confusing structure from which a public health system finally emerged in 1875. Chadwick may have had a blueprint ready for implementation in the 1840s, but in the circumstances of the time the painstaking accumulation of powers and functions was the only solution possible.[50]

This suggests that the historian should be far more concerned with the interrelationships of people, at all levels, their perceptions of the issues and how they are to be tackled, and with the 'desire' for individual freedom. When, however, the case was made: '. . . the state was prepared to embark on a journey which eventually led to a centralised administrative state'.[51] The culmination of this movement in public health was the formation of the Ministry of Health in 1919 at a time when public pressure was mounting and when medicine itself was showing positive results.[52]

Studies in social and public administration, and social policy have also contributed much to an understanding of political and administrative history, and particularly to health matters. Of particular relevance are Ruth Hodgkinson's study of poor law medical services in the years 1834-71, Jeanne Brand's research into the role played by the medical profession in the development of governmental action in public health during the period 1870-1912, and Rosemary Stevens' analysis of the specialisation process within medicine.[53] Bently Gilbert's detailed studies of the development of social policy in Britain also offers a mine of information for the social historian in medicine – particularly in the areas of the evolution of the school medical service and of National Health Insurance.[54] There are of course also many national and local studies on poor law administration, and on the development, in more recent times, of the National Health Service.[55] In the field of public administration, some interesting studies have been made of the development of Treasury control of the Civil Service, and particularly the appointment, and administration of medical staff.[56]

Intellectual and cultural history can be well seen through the social history of medicine. In a scientific sense, medicine may make progress, but an understanding must be reached of the modes and media by which new ideas percolate through different social strata, not only within the medical profession but also amongst the general population, and how these ideas are accepted or rejected. The impact of new technology and improved educational opportunities, which in themselves may create differences in level of knowledge and literacy, have to be taken into consideration: 'There is no reason to doubt, of course, the ability of the scientific method to solve each of the specific problems of disease by discovering causes and remedial procedures.'[57] Acceptance of the new knowledge and the creation of better health 'demands a kind of wisdom. . . which apprehends in all their complexities and subtleties the relation between living things and their total environment'.[58]

An excellent analysis of the concepts and perceptions of disease and health in sixteenth – and seventeenth-century England has emerged from the work of Keith Thomas.[59] He explains how 'the inadequacies of orthodox medical services left a large proportion of the population of Tudor and Stuart England dependent upon traditional folk medicine'.[60] This consisted essentially of

> . . . a mixture of common sensical remedies, based on the accumulated experience of nursing and midwifery combined with inherited lore about the healing properties of plants and minerals. But it also included certain types of ritual healing, in which prayers, charms or spells accompanied the medicine, or even formed the sole means of treatment. Magic healing of this kind might sometimes be attempted by the patient himself or a member of his family. More often it was the business of the cunning man, to whom the sufferer would have recourse, and to whom he would normally be expected to make some form of payment. Sometimes these wizards specialised in particular ailments; others claimed to be able to deal with them all.[61]

His explanation of the belief in magical healing lay in the beliefs of the curative power of the medieval Church, the survival of the concept of disease as a foreign element which could be transferred, and the thought that medical treatment was not understood by the ordinary man and was, therefore, magical. He studies the power of the royal touch and suggests that the power of suggestion was very strong:

> If anything the concept of psychosomatic disease was wider in the seventeenth century than it is now, for contemporary intellectuals

> tended to exaggerate the powers of the imagination. They thought that epidemics were likely to strike the fearful, and they believed that a pregnant women could shape the unborn foetus by her thoughts.[62]

This theme is taken up by Janet Blackman in the following essay in this collection – she considers the nature of the transmission of ideas from one generation to the next, and the acceptability and rejection of new scientific information. How were new ideas absorbed, re-interpreted or even rejected, not only at professional but also at lay or popular level? As Henry Miller, writing on medical literature, has noted: 'Knowledge is effective only if it can be widely understood and applied, and the function of the writer who communicates it successfully and accurately is second only to that of the discoverer.'[63]

It is to be hoped then that Janet Blackman's essay will draw attention to the important area of the history of the chain of medical ideas and their mode of communication, to both professional and lay recipients, and the roles of language, literacy and printing in this process. The development of railways and the penny post in the first half of the nineteenth century will need to be studied in relation to widening lines of communication. Thus as Sigerist has commented: '. . . we know much about the history of the great medical discoveries but very little on whether they were applied or to whom they were applied'.[64]

There has been much discussion regarding the development of a 'scientific community',[65] and studies in the history of science are starting to explore the pedigrees and genealogy of various scientific discoveries, together with the existence of influential groups.[66] Following on from Creighton's pioneering study of epidemics, detailed studies are now being made of the social history of particular diseases, and the development of knowledge in their control.[67] Another area in which it is possible to study transmission of medical views is in movements such as the Social Science Association, the campaigns to repeal the Contagious Diseases Act, together with the attempts to reduce prostitution and venereal disease, and the anti-compulsory vaccination struggles.[68] Although intrinsically important in themselves, historical studies of the Contagious Diseases Act have further value, since they can perhaps provide more information about attitudes to women and prostitutes than about venereal and other diseases. It remains evident, however, that at all times the patterns of health care provision have been dependent on the existing technology and the structure of society. It is thus possible for the social historian to see health problems such as the cholera epidemics, as agents of reform and to use health to seek explanation of the motives for institutional, social and administrative change.

The foregoing discussion has drawn attention to some of the extant literature which can be considered to be within the compass of the social history of medicine. It has of necessity been a selective review, and the aim has been to make a panoramic survey across a number of specialist areas.[69] Harold Perkin, however, has offered a timely reminder: 'The social historian must avoid the attempt to be everywhere at once. He must keep firmly in view his immediate goal, the understanding of the life of men in the past, in its setting of society and institutions.'[70] Thus the aim of a social history of medicine will be to seek an explanation of the internexus between health and disease, and society. To quote again from George Rosen:

> . . . to understand our society, the times in which we live, to be capable of playing an intelligent role in shaping our civilisation towards the future, we must have knowledge, not only of actions of the past, but of the mental struggles, the ideological and philosophical conflicts that preceded action, and of the groups and interests they represented.[71]

At this point it becomes important to focus on how the public used and viewed medical men, and their institutions and services. This will form one subject area of a historical sociology of medicine – another area which has been largely neglected:

> The social history of medicine. . . should include what the people who were most sadly involved thought and tried to do for themselves, and not only what was offered to them.[72]
> The unknown patient, too, deserves a monument and an account of how he fared and what commonly culled him down over the ages.[73]

This is to open up a new vista, and in particular a realisation that an individual's social status may have a profound effect on his perception of and attitude towards health, illness and doctors. As Rosen has written:

> . . . not only is disease related causally to the social and economic situation of the members of a given population, but the health care received also reflects the structure of a society, particularly its strat-

> ification and class divisions. Rank has its privileges in illness as in health. From antiquity to the present, the social class of patient has in various ways affected the medical transactions related to his illness.[74]

Studies in the sociology of medicine have recently drawn attention to the concept of the 'iceberg' of disease – unrecognised disease, and disease which if recognised by the individual is not brought to the doctor for treatment. Processes in the progress of patienthood are considered later in this essay, but it should be noted that as far back as 1936 Sigerist was drawing attention to the importance of the 'iceberg' concept for the social historian: '. . . medicine is not only what the physician does. The majority of all cases of illness – the minor ailments – are never seen by a physician. They are treated by the patient himself or by his relatives.'[75] The social history of medicine therefore concerns itself precisely with the relationships between doctors, dentists, or allied health personnel and patients, and between health professionals and society. To quote again from Sigerist:

> We have to study the position of physician and patient in a given society, their attitude towards the human body, the valuation of health, and disease at a given time. The scientific standard of a physician alone does not make him efficient. Society has to be ready and willing to accept his advice.[76]

In recent years, in both England and the United States, there has developed an increasing interest in the sociology of medicine. In this country the line of development has been predominantly pragmatic – an attempt to explain, with suitable statistical detail, reasons for the public's current failure to make optimum use of existing health care facilities. Of late, however, there has been evolving a more theoretical sense in which sociological knowledge of health concerns is advanced not just as a response to pressing health service deficiencies but more as part of an attempt to explain social structure and social behaviour. Except for the publications reviewed immediately below (from what may be termed the 'Leicester School'), there has been little work in the historical sociology of medicine, and the prime focus of attention has been on current phenomena and deficiencies.

Holloway has explained some of the problems facing the relationship between sociology and history. He sees the historian as being engaged in tracing a chronological sequence of past events and in showing how certain events led on to others, and the sociologist as interested in functional relationships which exist between analytically separable elements in societies.[78] The sociologist is then, *inter alia,* particularly interested in studying (a) relationships between different individuals and groups in society, (b) how these relationships are organised into institutions, (c) how these institutions are interrelated, and (d) the mechanisms by which they are changing. Thus as Bryan Wilson has suggested: '. . . the sociologist is less interested in chronological sequence than in processual sequence',[79] i.e. he is more interested in 'stages' than 'periods'. The sociologist approaches medicine as a case illustration of an explicit conceptual model, and studies such topics as roles, functions, relationships, beliefs, professionalisation, status and social structure.

Holloway has attempted a reinterpretation of the Apothecaries Act of 1815,[80] and further sought a sociological explanation of changes within medical education during the period 1830-58. As he himself notes:

> . . . it is possible neither to describe these changes adequately except within the context of other changes in social structure. The explanatory model used. . . is one which emphasises the interrelationship and interaction of various systems in a society undergoing a process of social change. Briefly, the four systems to be considered are, the system of medical education, the corpus of medical knowledge, the social structure of the medical profession, and the social structure of the wider society.[81]

As he shows, during the period 1830-58 medical knowledge became more scientific, medical education more systematic and the medical profession more unified.

The stimulus provided by Holloway for a historical review of medicine using sociological analysis has let to to further studies by his colleagues, Ivan Waddington and Nicholas Jewson. Waddington has studied attempts to reform the Royal College of Physicians in the years 1767-71. He focuses on the social basis of the struggle and on the attempts at usurption of role, and argues that the social origins of reform were affected by the introduction of a new type of medical practitioner who cut across the tripartite division of physicians, surgeons and apothecaries. In another paper he describes the evolution of a system of medical ethics, and argues that it developed more in the context of relationships between practitioners themselves, than between practitioners and their clients – thereby challenging accepted concepts of professional ethics.[82] Above all it is therefore important to study changing relationships between practitioners, as for example Waddington himself does in his essay, in this collection, on the relationships between consultants and general practitioners.

Waddington has also outlined some of the salient characteristics of the social organisation within hospitals in nineteenth-century Paris, and shown how the internal social structure facilitated changes in the structure of medical knowledge. Of particular relevance was the change from client to doctor-control of medical transactions within the hospital scene.[83] Waddington's colleague, Jewson, has described aspects of medical knowledge and the patronage system in eighteenth-century England. He examines the relationship and interaction between physicians and their aristocratic patients, and suggests effects of client-control on medical innovation and beliefs, and the development of scientific medicine.[84]

As indicated above, the committed interest of sociologists in Britain in attempting to analyse structures and processes in health care is a recent phenomenon. The studies by Holloway, Waddington and Jewson remain almost the sum total of effort in a historical sociology of medicine. Abel-Smith, Richards and Donnison, however, have used sociological concepts in their historical descriptions of the pathway towards professional status, governmental legitimisation and state recognition taken by nursing, dentistry and midwifery.[85]

The bulk of medical sociological research in Britain has thus concerned examinations of contemporary society. Detailed explanation and interpretation of present behaviour and attitudes can, however, often only be possible following a consideration of their antecedents. Studies in the field of dental health serve as a prime example of this point. During the mid-1960s the first empirical studies of public use of dentists and of attitudes to dental health and dental care were undertaken in this country, and a correlation was made between what lay individuals thought about their dental conditions and what dentists found on examination. The investigators reported revealing differences, particularly concerning peridontal and gum health. Explanation for current knowledge, beliefs and practices was sought by attempting to open up a historical sociology of dentistry.[86] This has involved consideration of the fact that dentistry is above all else a social activity, involving a dynamic and changing relationship between a provider and consumer of dental care. As Freidson has argued,[87] many studies of the professional process have omitted any reference to the role of the patient, and the nature of medical practice is seen as determined largely by the practitioner's relationship to his colleagues, and their institutions, and by his profession's relationship with the State. It is very clear that dental practice cannot exist without patients, who have ideas about what they want, and these may differ markedly from those supposedly held by the dentist they consult. Thus dentists, like doctors, practise not merely in surgeries but also in a social environment, which helps to shape and mould behaviour and attitudes. In attempting to explain what is transacted in a dental surgery, it is important both to chronicle what dental professionals believe and do, and, perhaps more importantly, also to understand public reaction to available treatment and prophylactic practices. At present, as in the field of medical care, there are more questions than answers: How did the general public view dentists and the need for dental care? what processes did a potential patient go through before arriving at a particular dentist's surgery? what factors were important in recruitment to the dental profession? how far was dental behaviour class-related, and were there differing class-perceptions of the need and demand for dental care? what image of dentistry was transmitted by a visit to a dentist? These are some of the important questions for a historical sociology of dentistry to answer. Only by attempting to study the past will it be possible to offer a total examination of present practice and beliefs – thus the utilitarian rather than esoteric function of a historical approach. Even if answers to such questions as those posed above are not immediately forthcoming, it is important that the questions in these and parallel areas be put, for the social dimension to the development of health services has been sadly neglected. Very few of the standard histories of medicine or dentistry have had either any substantial regard for the consumers of care, or any awareness of social structural differences in knowledge, beliefs, attitudes and behaviour. By its very existence a historical sociology of medicine can illuminate new areas – for historians, sociologists and doctors there are many pay-offs, provided that it is understood that changes in attitudes to illness, caring behaviour and treatment patterns have themselves taken place in a changing milieu and socio-cultural system.

Even if the sociology of medicine has largely ignored the historical perspective there are nonetheless some important concepts from current research which may have considerable bearing upon explanations of past developments in medical care, and may therefore be of importance to the social historian of medicine.[88] Indeed, in Britain and in recent years following the publication of the (Todd) Report of the Royal Commission on Medical Education in 1968, medical sociology has figured as a larger component in medical school curricula, and has been spawning its own textbooks.[89] Two main strands of development may be discerned – sociology *of* medicine which uses medical settings to study the organisational structure, role-relationships, value systems, attitudes and systems of behaviour, and sociology *in* medicine, which applies this knowledge to solve medical problems.[90]

In describing the setting in which social policy has developed Richard Titmuss has suggested that '. . . we have to see it in the context of a particular set of circumstances, a given society and culture, and a more or less specified period of historical time'[91] – that is to say not in a social vacuum, in which individuals do not exist merely as a mass of separate identities but as part of a social system. His comments also relate to the development of medical care and health service policy. Sociological information about the following areas was, he suggested, of prime importance – knowledge of population changes, past and present, and predicted for the future; the family as an institution and the position of women; social stratification and the concepts of class, caste, status and mobility; social change and the effects of industrialisation, urbanisation, and social conditions; the political structure; the work ethic and the sociology of industrial relations; minority groups and racial prejudice, and social control, conformity and deviance.[92] It is clear then that sociology has much to contribute to an understanding of the historical development of medicine and medical services. From the vast and growing literature in the field of medical sociology six areas have been selected for further comment – the role of the sick person, utilisation of medical services, the doctor-patient relationship, the professionalisation process, the role of the hospital and of medical institutions, and studies of innovation processes.

An important area for medical sociological research has concerned the role and status of the sick person. Increasingly it has been realised that to be sick is a social phenomenon, and affects one's relationship to others. That the sick person occupies a special position in the social structure has been recognised for some years. Sigerist and Henderson, in 1929 and 1935 respectively, supplied the foundation upon which Parsons in 1951 elaborated in the concept of the 'sick role'.[93] Much critical discussion has followed, and this has prompted development of further concepts of health, illness, normality and deviance. As David Mechanic has explained, there is clearly something about a person's social position that influences his perception and interpretation of symptoms, and the way he reacts to them. Mechanic has developed the concept of illness behaviour, defined as 'the way in which given symptoms may be differentially perceived, evaluated and acted (or not acted) upon by different persons'.[94]

Elsewhere he has explored the way in which various contexts bring about different and sometimes conflicting definitions of illness and social disability, as well as varied and modified role obligations on the part of the sick person.[95] It is, however, clear, from consideration of the 'iceberg' concept mentioned above, that not all organically sick persons define themselves as ill and come under medical scrutiny. Koos' pioneering study has shown that the same symptoms and complaints can be differentially interpreted by laymen in different social strata and that factors other than strictly medical ones are important in defining illness.[96] Thus a professional's view of illness, which has been moulded by clinical experience may differ markedly from a patient's view, which has been largely influenced by the need to cope with a particular problem and by his understanding of the nature of the problem. As Twaddle has noted, 'only recently has illness become an event for which explanations could be sought outside the realm of biology and medicine'.[97]

Mechanic has listed some of the correlates which sociologists have suggested affect response to illness: (a) visibility, recognisability, and salience of symptoms, (b) severity of symptoms, (c) extent to which symptoms disrupt normal activity, (d) frequency, persistence, and recurrence of symptoms, (e) tolerance threshold, (f) available information, knowledge and cultural assumptions, (g) denial tendencies, (h) competing needs, (i) competing interpretations, and (j) availability and cost of treatment.[98] To these might be added situational factors which make it more or less difficult to seek care (i.e. problems of distance, transport and time) and faith in the medical care team to provide easy and lasting solutions. Perception and recognition of a need for medical care does not necessarily mean a formal consultation with a doctor. Resort to self-medication is an important area to which sociological research has drawn attention.[99] What has been the traditional role assigned to self-medication? Study of advertisements for patent medicines, pills and ointments will permit an examination of this area.

At some point individuals translate their felt need for medical attention into utilisation of a doctor's services. A plethora of research studies in many countries has focused on reasons for use of medical and dental services, and on stages in and pathways to medical care.[100] Suchman and Zola have developed notions of decision-making points and factors influencing the decision to seek medical aid. Suchman has also drawn attention to the structure of social groups and health orientations or value systems, and their relationship to use of health services.[101] Evidence from many studies points to the importance of socio-demographic factors in combining to produce a differential use of health services. The roles of education, occupation, location, residence, family size, religion, age and sex have been well documented. Research has also concerned the relationship between beliefs and attitudes, and behaviour, and there has been much debate on whether behaviour determines beliefs and attitudes, or vice versa. Another important concern has been that of the role of what Freidson has termed the 'lay referral system', that is, the role of the network of personal influence, involving kinship and friendship patterns, along which a patient travels on his way to see the doctor.[102] This is of course to ask who in the family is or was the decision-maker with regard to health matters, and to question a patient's relationship with not only registered doctors, but also with competing diagnostic and therapeutic systems – i.e. quacks and unregistered practitioners.

Much of this research has concerned use of preventive medicine, and has implied the existence of some rational decision: in the nineteenth century, however, doctors were consulted for more obvious disease. Economic factors may have been important – there has, however, been little emphasis on attempting, even from available records, to define use of nineteenth-century medical facilities. Holloway has suggested that demand for medical care in the early nineteenth century came entirely from the middle and upper classes, and was dependent more on economic factors than attitudes or beliefs.[103] It is clear, however, that a health consciousness developed in the later years of the century, particularly amongst aspiring and middle-class people. What were the roots of this development, and how far is it possible to chart and describe its progress, particularly in relation to the concept of the Protestant Ethic? How far were knowledge and behaviour related? As people became more literate and more knowledgeable about health, what effects were there on use of medical services? In making these brief remarks on utilisation behaviour, the intention, once again, has not been to be comprehensive, but rather to open up an area which has lacked a multi-disciplinary approach, and has been largely ignored in historical research.

People seeking medical care and health practitioners may be seen as two components of an interacting social system. There has been much comment from the medical profession concerning the forum in which sick persons consult them. Increasingly there has, however, developed a deeper knowledge of how patients regard doctors and the therapeutic relationship.[104] Important in this respect has been a growing awareness of the patient as a participant rather than merely a recipient of care.[105] Stimson and Webb have recently undertaken an analysis of the process of consultation with a doctor, and considered not just what occurs at the point of contact itself but also the antecedents and postcripts.[106] The importance of the doctor-patient interaction and relationship has been stressed by many researchers.[107] Szasz and Hollender conceived of a basic model of the relationship, involving three types of doctor-patient interaction: activity-passivity (in which the doctor is in absolute control); guidance-co-operation (in which the patient is expected to do what he is told), and mutual participation. These relationships will transpire depending on the disease the patient has, and the therapy considered appropriate by the doctor. As Freidson has pointed out, there are, however, other types of relationship – namely co-operation-guidance (where the doctor co-operates and the patient guides) and passivity-activity (where the patient is active).[108] But how much do patients follow doctors' recommendations? Studies of the role of compliance reveal interesting differences dependent on different diseases.[109] What, however, of the historical development of the doctor-patient relationship? Clearly there have been changes over time in relation to the typology suggested above, particularly as doctors during the nineteenth century assumed a more dominant role. In short, who treated whom for what, and what was the nature and duration of the doctor-patient relationship?

A particularly pertinent area of sociological research has concerned the professional status of medicine. Over the years there has been considerable debate regarding the concept of professional status, and it is evident that no absolute definitions exist.[110] Essential attributes would seem to include pre-empting, institutionalizing, legitimising, and autonomising elements. Freidson provides a particularly revealing analysis of medicine's collective struggle for professional status. Waddington's analyses of internal struggles between physicians, surgeons and apothecaries serve as a reminder of warring factions within medicine itself, and prompt a consideration of the process whereby specialisation and subprofessionalisation occur. Earlier sections of this essay have alluded to professionalisation in medicine, and it is clear that this is one area where cross-fertilisation between sociologists and historians has already taken place. Nevertheless as Freidson has commented:

> The most conventional investigations which historians have most often performed are addressed to the state of scientific medical

> knowledge in a particular period, the biographies of medical men, and the circumstances surrounding a particular scientific discovery.[111]

He noted the existence of much primary and secondary source material, and added his hope that 'Sociologists, if not historians, may make more use of such material in the future.'[112] Important for any deeper understanding of the social development of medicine as a profession will be an analysis of recruitment – who entered medical school, and from what backgrounds did entrants come?

A further area of sociological commitment concerns the hospital as a bureaucratic and institutional structure in which medical care is practised.[113] The hospital is a forum for interactions between patients, doctors, nurses, administrators and others – it is then a complex administrative setting. Few of the hospital histories have provided any insight into the interactions and struggles which took place inside the institutions. It is evident that over the years there have been important changes in the power groups: ecclesiastics, social philanthropists, medical staff and administrators have all had roles to play. There is also an important need to identify the circumstances, interests and values influencing the development of hospitals. Human relations and organisational behaviour have formed two key areas for sociological study of hospital practices – again there has been little use made of these approaches in a historical setting.

Mankind inherits vast amounts of knowledge from his predecessors, adds to this storehouse a small amount of new knowledge, and passes it on to his descendants. How is the new knowledge diffused and disseminated? Sociological studies of innovations, particularly new drugs and new health practices, provide a particularly insightful area. Diffusion research has been concerned with the flow of new ideas, values and practices. How are they imported into the social system, and what factors determine the rate of spread? A particularly revealing study, and one which has many historical implications, was undertaken by Coleman, Katz and Menzel.[114] They studied a new drug, and its acceptance through time and among doctors. They underlined the role of links and contacts – the more deeply integrated a doctor was in his local medical community, the more likely he was to be an early user of the drug. Parallel with this there has developed what has been termed the 'two-step flow of communication' i.e. ideas flow via opinion leaders to less active sections of the public. Who were the opinion leaders in the medical profession? Further work by E.S. Rogers has considered stages

In the adoption process: awareness, information, evaluation, trial and adoption. Together with A.E. Niehoff he has suggested some of the important characteristics of innovators and recipients.[115] There is considerable scope for the application of concepts from this area to a study of the innovation of new medical practices, and of factors which influenced their diffusion and adoption.

Closely related to the need for a wider understanding of sociological concepts will be a parallel need for an awareness of anthropological and cultural components of health, disease and medicine. Pellegrino has stressed the importance of culture: 'The medical behaviour of individuals and groups is incomprehensible apart from general cultural history.'[116] Indeed, in his study of science, medicine and reform in the seventeenth century, Charles Webster has underlined the impossibility of understanding the scientific outlook of society without reference to the more general context of prevailing beliefs and values.[117]

Much recent work has stressed how cultural, moral and religious views underline the explanation of illness.[118] In recent times the nature and influence of a conflict in cultural values, and thereby often a failure in health service innovation and the introduction of unanticipated effects, have been well documented. In studies of technological change it is possible to point to a failure to understand the relationship between, on the one hand, traditional values, beliefs and behaviour, and, on the other, social, cultural, religious and ethnic structures and systems.[119] In particular, Paul's monograph catalogues a series of intervention studies in widely different cultural settings, and provides overwhelming evidence of the need for successful health innovations to take account of existing community organisation, local customs, values, symbols, totems, taboos, and religious beliefs. Such studies document a failure to weave scientifically-tested discoveries into a fabric of daily life.[120] Indeed the essence of such studies is to underline the magnitude of gaps between the interpretations of medical personnel, and of the populations they serve. Thus cultural blinkers may often prevent a true comprehension of the needs and desires of people, and lead to an insensitivity as regards social and cultural consequences. An understanding of these areas will facilitate a deeper analysis of the apparent frustration felt, over the years, by many health professionals following a lack of response by the public to exhortations that they should change their health and illness behaviour. Such behaviour cannot be seen in isolation, and indeed often is only explicable in terms of a total cultural configuration.

Awareness of cultural concepts will also encourage a more perceptive study of the roles played by witchcraft and sorcery, by traditional healers and quack practitioners, and by folk remedies.[121] Anthropological viewpoints have been largely neglected in the history of medicine – indeed, some twenty-five years ago, one American anthropologist, Monica Wilson, asked what were the social conditions in England which produced witchcraft beliefs, and what were the causes and effects of declines in such beliefs. She concluded her paper with this hope: 'I long to read an adequate analysis of this problem. . .by a social historian aware of anthropological theory.'[122] The perceptive studies by Alan Macfarlane and Keith Thomas bear evidence of a growing awareness of the relationship between health, history and anthropology, but also pose important questions for future research – for example, how far is a belief in witchcraft or in folk medicine affected by changes in societal organisation and kinship systems, and by increases in literacy, knowledge, urbanisation and industrialisation?

Some recent developments in social history and the sociology of medicine have been reviewed in the preceding pages. In seeking to promote and realign a social history of medicine this selective review has not attempted to cover every possible approach but merely to indicate the range and scope of avenues for future development. The suggestion has been made that undue emphasis has hitherto been focused on the providers of medical care, i.e. doctors, and that as a result there has been a corresponding neglect of consideration of lay and patient viewpoints. Furthermore there has been little attempt at explaining how advances in scientific medicine were disseminated amongst both the medical profession and the general public, and how changing concepts of and attitudes towards diseases, such as mental illness and insanity, and venereal diseases, have shaped and themselves been moulded by changes in provision of services.[123] Changing 'power relationships' between doctors and patients have affected medical practice – it will be the task of a social history of medicine to define more precisely how 'patient power' has developed. Another important area which awaits detailed analysis is that of societal attitudes and practices regarding segregation, certification and internment of sick individuals – what are the roots of the move to cut back on institutional and custodial treatment, and to advocate community care? Yet a further area concerns the study of the social geography of the spread of disease, and of the dissemination of new medical ideas and practices. Not only how far did lay beliefs differ, but what has been the effect of the distribution of medical manpower, schooled in different medical centres and cultures, over the country as a whole? As George Rosen has noted 'one of the next assignments for medical historians is to put disease on the map'.[124] The itinerary and contours of many medical and lay beliefs, attitudes and behaviours still remain uncharted.

In this short essay it is not intended to set any precise parameters to what specific areas fall within the precinct of a social history of medicine. What has been stressed, however, has been the need for a closer liaison between and awareness of the viewpoints of history, sociology and medicine. The Society for the Social History of Medicine has been instituted to develop these very ideals, and to draw together the various threads. It has sought to range far and wide in its coverage – as some titles of recently delivered papers suggest: 'A Centennial Retrospective View of the Royal Sanitary Commission', 'The Medical Officer of Health 1848-1973, 'Medicine and Pharmacy in French Political Prints', 'Chance or Choice: Eugenics from Frank to Galton', 'Water Cure Therapeutics 1840-1870', 'Child Health and Diet in the Nineteenth Century', 'Morals and Molars – Physical Deterioration and the Beginnings of the School Dental Service', 'State, Church, Charity and Smallpox: Mexico 1797-1798', 'The Reality of Anticontagionism – Theories of Epidemic Disease in the Early Nineteenth Century', and 'The Crisis of Subsistence and Health of the Puritan Revolution'. Each of these papers has sparked off a dialogue between interested disciplines, and it is to be hoped that the papers in this collection will prompt a similar response.

This essay has reiterated the need for a continuing introduction of a social perspective in studying the history of medicine – a need which Sigerist stressed in his many writings. Indeed one of the many obituary tributes about his work elaborated on the new approach which he pioneered:

> . . . medical history so far had been largely the history of great doctors or medical scientists. But nobody had as yet written the history of the patient, the history of the attitudes towards medicine in an ever-changing world, the history of the appreciation of medical services, in short the history of medicine as dependent upon the specific spirit of a given age.[125]

Poynter was another to note the new influences:

> (Sigerist's) insistence that the patient should share the centre of the stage with the physician did much to liberate medical history from the narrow confines of literary history, and to integrate the history of medicine with social history, both being in his opinion,

sociological studies.[126]

Thus the social importances have been stressed, and it has been recognised, in some quarters at least, that 'in approaching the History of Medicine one is very prone to lay too much emphasis on the great discoveries and inventions, or dramatic episodes'.[127] For one historian, however, the history of medicine was a sterile field: '. . . most of it was mere antiquarianism, relieved by hagiographies of outstanding physicians'.[128] He saw a new future ahead: '. . . the social historian of medicine is the observer and interpreter of centuries of medical activity in various social contexts'.[129]

Is it, however, possible to say that much progress has been made since Sigerist's day? It is to be hoped that the areas selectively reviewed in this paper will demonstrate some of the scholarly advances made by social historians and sociologists in seeking a deeper explanation of the role of health, disease and medicine in society. Their studies have been very much individual efforts, and there has hardly been any codification of relevant data. Theories and findings of separate investigations have all too seldom been linked together, or applied in other studies – there is thus need for a fusion of the historical, sociological and medical approaches towards an institutionalisation of a social history of medicine. However, as Lester King has warned:

> . . . advance does not come from the mere combination of two or more disciplines. A sociologist and a historian and a physician, placed together, will not create a social history of medicine. There must be a synthesis. Masses of facts, derived from separate disciplines, and placed side by side, accomplish nothing. Some spark of new insight must place these data into meaningful relationship – and 'insight' is merely another word for 'interpretation'. Progress comes when an investigator in one field perceives the relevance of data in another field. Furthermore he must have enough knowledge of both fields to make his insight meaningful and appealing to others.[130]

It is to be hoped that the essays in this book will show some evidence of this new insight, and point the way to future endeavour. It will be important for existing judgements to be examined and interpreted, for from such analyses may come a deeper and more perceptive understanding of the social role of health and illness, and of social aspects to the organisation of the medical profession and medical services.

Thomas McKeown, at the inaugural meeting of the Society for the Social History of Medicine, chose as the title of his paper: 'A Sociological Approach to the History of Medicine', and derived his focus from Sigerist's belief that 'the sociological approach to the history of medicine not only gives us a better understanding of the past but can also help in planning the future'. On this interpretation McKeown believed that if social history, as Trevelyan quipped, was history with the politics left out, then the social history of medicine was medical history with the public interest put in.[131] This book is intended to supplement this philosophy, by urging that the social history of medicine is both medical history with people, patients and society put in, and also the history of people, patients and society with medicine put in.

The proposition then is for a social history of medicine which starts not from an iatrocentric but from a sociocentric viewpoint. In the contemporary idiom Ivan Illich is a harsh critic of clinical iatrogenesis; he has argued for an understanding of social and structural elements, for, as he comments 'man, unmodified by a particular place and companionship, simply does not exist'.[132] He questions the need for what Freidson, in his penetrating analysis of the medical profession, has termed 'professional dominance':[133]

> When dependence on the professional management of pain, sickness and death grows beyond a certain point, the healing power in sickness, patience, in suffering and fortitude in the face of death must decline. These three regressions are symptoms of third-level iatrogenesis: their combined outcome is Medical Nemesis.[134]

A social history of medicine can seek to explain how roles, and relationships between doctors and patients have changed, and trace the influence exerted not only by medicine upon society, but also by society on medicine.

This exploratory essay, which has drawn heavily on but two aspects of a wider thematic approach, namely Britain and the nineteenth century (it will be important to stress the development of studies in other countries, or over other centuries), concludes with some penetrating comments made by George Rosen at the Third International Conference on Social Science and Medicine, held at Elsinore in August 1972:

> Attention to the maintenance of good health, and care of the sick and disabled, have been an element of group life throughout recorded

history and in all likelihood long before. As a social activity such care is interlocked in various ways and in differing degree with the structure of group living of which it is a part – with the family, religion, the economy, government, the value system and other elements. Furthermore, not only is the structure of health care inseparable from the general organisation of society, but its reality cannot be fully discovered from static, cross-sectional analysis. Like any other social institution, medicine experiences both continuity and change, so that its past differs from its present, and it will be something different in the future, and yet for good or for ill what happened in the past influences the present and the future.

This dynamic aspect is the history of health care. History derives from challenges experienced by various groups of people, and the ways in which they respond to them. The result is a variety of actions and reactions under different circumstances and often under widely divergent ideological and emotional climates. Yet those actions and reactions have in one way or another brought us to the present. Institutions, patterns of behaviour, systems of ideas – all have developed from something which was there before. Attitudes towards illness, theories of disease, arrangements for the care of affected individuals, modes of treatment and the practitioners who provide them – all illustrate this truism which is too often overlooked. Historical analysis makes it possible to penetrate past social structures and the changes they have experienced in the course of time so as to illuminate our understanding of the process of development which has led to the present, thus providing meaning and significance not to be found in a study restricted solely to a contemporary segment. This is a basic function of medical history, to lay bare the origins of medical institutions, their organisation, ideas and operation, and to explain their significance. The translation of medical and other values is likewise historically conditioned, and historical studies can throw light on this aspect as well. An account of how it came into existence will reveal the prevailing structure of health services in sharp perspective and highlight its dynamics.

Medicine as a social activity undertaken within the context of human need and group life develops institutional forms through which ideas and practices are carried out by members of an organised society, characterised by division of labour and specialisation of function. Viewed in these terms, medicine, or health care, can be studied by any means available for the investigation of social institutions. In fact, social scientists (sociologists, psychologists, anthropologists, economists) have been making such studies, and their efforts have to a greater or lesser degree employed historical approaches and materials. In the light of this situation which is likely to expand, what can and should be the relations between history and the social sciences in the field of our common interest, health in its various aspects? No social science is a totally self-contained system, and each has areas and facets that border on other disciplines including historical studies.[135]

A social history of medicine, using the above ideas as its text, will be of the utmost value, not only for an explanation of health and illness behaviour in past societies but in helping to understand contemporary actions and reactions. Thereby it will serve history, sociology and medicine.

Notes

1. E.H. Carr, *What is History?,* London, 1961, p.60. See also amongst others T.H. Marshall, 'Max Weber: an intellectual portrait by Reinhard Bendix: review article', *British Journal of Sociology, 12,* 1961, 184-8; Asa Briggs, 'Sociology and history', in A.T. Welford (ed.), *Society. Problems and Methods of Study,* London, 1962, pp.91-8, and his 'History and society', in N. MacKenzie (ed.), *A Guide to the Social Sciences,* London, 1966, pp.33-53; S.W.F. Holloway, 'Sociology and history', *History, 48,* 1963, 154-80; S.M. Lipset and R. Hofstadter, *Sociology and History: Methods,* New York, 1968, and B.R. Wilson, 'Sociological methods in the study of history', *Transactions of the Royal Historical Society, 21,* 1971, 101-18. Few however, can have been as provocatively succinct as Donald G. MacRae, who saw sociology as 'history with the hard work left out', and history as 'sociology with the brains left out' – see his 'Some sociological perspectives' in International Sociological Association, *Transactions of the Third World Conference of Sociology,* vol. 8, London, 1956, p. 302.
2. George Rosen, 'Social variables and health in an urban environment: the case of the Victorian city', *Clio Medica, 8,* 1973, 1.
3. George Rosen, 'The new history of medicine: a review', *Journal of the History of Medicine and Allied Sciences, 6,* 1951, 519-20.
4. See F.H. Garrison, *An Introduction to the History of Medicine,* Philadelphia, 1913; Sir William Osler, *The Evolution of Modern Medicine,* New Haven, 1921; C.G. Cumston, *An Introduction to the History of Medicine,* London, 1926; C. Singer, *A Short History of Medicine,* Oxford, 1928 (and a second edition by Singer and E.A. Underwood, Oxford 1962); D. Guthrie, *A History of Medicine,* London 1945; A. Castiglioni, *A History of Medicine* (trans. and ed. by E.B. Krumbhaar), New York, 1947, and A. Pazzini, *Storia della Medicina,* 2 vols., Milan, 1947. For a historiographical review of the field, and one which in twenty-one collected essays strangely neglect social history and medical sociology as specialist subject areas, see Edwin Clarke (ed.), *Modern Methods in the History of Medicine,* London, 1971.

5. George Rosen, 'Levels of integration in medical historiography: a review', *Journal of the History of Medicine and Allied Sciences, 4,* 1949, 465.
6. Henry E. Sigerist, 'The history of medicine and the history of science', *Bulletin of the History of Medicine, 4,* 1936, 5.
7. Charles F. Mullett, 'Medical history: some problems and opportunities', *Journal of the History of Medicine and Allied Sciences, 1,* 1946, 190.
8. *Ibid.*, 204
9. *Ibid.*
10. *Ibid.*
11. On the plague see for example J.F.D. Shrewsbury, *A History of the Bubonic Plague in the British Isles,* Cambridge, 1970. On the implications of cholera especially in the European context, see L. Chevalier, *Le Cholera. La Premiere Epidemie du XIXe Siecle,* La Roche-sur-Yon, 1958. For an account of cholera epidemics in this country see N. Longmate, *King Cholera,* London, 1966.
12. George Rosen, *The History of Miners' Disease,* New York, 1943.
13. *Ibid.,* p.ix. On the development of occupational and industrial medicine in nineteenth-century England, see W.R. Lee, 'Robert Baker: the first doctor in the factory department', *British Journal of Industrial Medicine, 21,* 1964, 85-93 and 167-79; his 'An anatomy of occupational medicine', *British Journal of Industrial Medicine, 30,* 1973, 111-17, and his 'Emergence of occupational medicine in Victorian times', *British Journal of Industrial Medicine, 30,* 1973, 118-24; Michael E. Rose, 'The doctor and the industrial revolution', *British Journal of Industrial Medicine, 28,* 1971, 22-6, and James A. Smiley, 'Some aspects of the early evolution of the appointed factory doctor service', *British Journal of Industrial Medicine, 28,* 1971, 315-22.
14. William Ashworth, *The Genesis of Modern British Town Planning,* London, 1954, and Asa Briggs, *History of Birmingham. Borough and City. 1865-1938, 1938,* vol. II, London, 1952, On the history of public health see W.M. Frazer, *The History of English Public Health, 1834-1939,* London, 1950; C.F. Brockington, *Public Health in the Nineteenth Century,* London 1965. For a survey taking a wide-angle lens, and indicative of the multi-sided approach advocated in this paper, see George Rosen, *A History of Public Health,* New York, 1958.
15. R.A. Lewis, *Edwin Chadwick and the Public Health Movement, 1832-1854,* London, 1952; S.E. Finer, *The Life and Times of Edwin Chadwick,* London, 1952; and Royston Lambert, *Sir John Simon, 1816-1904, and English Social Administration,* London, 1963.
16. E.J. Hobsbawm, 'From social history to the history of society', in M. Flinn and T.C. Smout (eds.), *Essays in Social History,* London 1947, p. 5.
17. *Ibid.,* p. 9.
18. Carr, *op. cit.,* p. 9.
19. See for example Harold Perkin, *The Origins of Modern English Society, 1780-1880,* London, 1969, and Asa Briggs, *Victorian People,* London, 1954; his *The Age of Improvement,* London, 1959; and his *Victorian Cities,* London, 1963.
20. D.S. Landes and C. Tilly (eds.), *History as a Social Science,* Englewood Cliffs, New Jersey, 1971, p.5.
21. Hobsbawm, *op. cit.,* p. 6.
22. Neil J. Smelser, *Social Change in the Industrial Revolution: an Application of Theory to the Lancashire Cotton Industry, 1770-1840,* London, 1959, and Michael Anderson, *Family Structure in Nineteenth Century Lancashire,* London, 1971.

23. David C. McClelland, *The Achieving Society*, New York, 1961, and Everett E. Hagen, *On the Theory of Social Change*, London, 1964.
24. Carr, *op. cit.*, p. 17.
25. Asa Briggs, 'The study of the history of education', *History of Education, 1*, 1972, 5-22
26. J.B. Bertrand, *A Historical Relation of the Plague at Marseilles in the Year 1720* (translated by Anne Plumptre), London 1805, (reprinted London, 1973, with an introduction by J.N. Biraben). A wide literature may be cited in the field of local studies of health and health services: three prime areas concern local hospitals, and their statistics and systems of administration, medical records from general practice, and health departments. Symptomatic of much work in these areas are W.B. Howie's studies of the Salop Infirmary – 'The administration of an eighteenth century provincial hospital (1747-1830)', *Medical History, 5*, 1961, 34-55 and his 'Finance and supply in an eighteenth century hospital', *Medical History, 7*, 1963, 126-46 (for a bibliography on voluntary hospitals see John Woodward, *To Do the Sick No Harm. A Study of the British Voluntary Hospital System to 1875*, London and Boston, 1974, pp. 202-14); R.M.S. McConaghey , 'Medical records of Dartmouth 1425-1887', *Medical History, 4*, 1960, 91-109; A.K. Chalmers, *The Health of Glasgow, 1818-1925*, Glasgow, 1930, and Sir Alexander MacGregor, *Public Health in Glasgow*, Edinburgh, 1967. The reorganisation of the National Health Service in 1974 has occasioned a number of studies of local health departments – see B.M. Barrows, *A County and Its Health – A History of the Development of the West Riding Health Services 1889-1974* Wakefield, 1974; and H.P. Tait, *A Doctor and Two Policemen, the History of Edinburgh Health Department 1862-1974*, Edinburgh, 1974.
27. Bertrand (Biraben introduction), p. i.
28. *Ibid.*, p. ii.
29. *Ibid.*, pp. ii-iii.
30. *Ibid.*, p. v. Biraben, as one of the foremost of contemporary French demographers, has made a general study of the plague in the history of population. See his *Les Hommes et la Peste*, Paris, 1974, vol. I, and his paper with Jacques le Goff, 'La peste dans le haut moyen age' in *Annales: E.S.C., 24*, 1969, 1484-510 (reprinted and translated in R. Forster and O. Ranum (eds.), *Biology of Man in History*, Baltimore and London, 1975). For a recent study of the effects of the plague in Colchester, which stresses the need for further local studies see I.G. Doolittle, 'The effects of the plague on a provincial town in the sixteenth and seventeenth centuries', *Medical History, 19*, 1975, 333-41.
31. R.F. Berkhofer, *A Behavioural Approach to Historical Analysis*, New York and London, 1969, pp. 252-3.
32. John D. Post, 'Famine mortality and epidemic disease in the process of modernisation', *Economic History Review, 29*, 1976, 14-37. For a fascinating recreation of the world of the rural sick in France during the period 1774-95 see Jean-Pierre Peter's study of the archives of the Societe Royale de Medicine, 'Malades et maladies a la fin du XVIIIe siecle', *Annales: E.S.C., 22.* 1967, 711-51 (reprinted and translated in Forster and Ranum, *op. cit.*)
33. Post, *op. cit.*, p. 31. For a particular study of an outbreak in Italy in the seventeenth century see C. Cipolla, *Cristofano and the Plague*, Berkeley, California, 1973. His preface describes the book's objective: '. . . there are numerous histories of plague and of individual epidemics – local or widespread. However, this is not – nor does it set out to be – a history of a

plague in the traditional sense. At least in the intention of its author, what follows is rather the story of a small land, caught in a tragic mess – and of the way in which they reacted to it. They were men – with their virtues and their defects. There were no saints. Some however responded much better than others. The tragedy gave the opportunity to some to show initiative, courage, civic sense, humanity. But at the same time tragedy and death were not enough to eliminate from the hearts of people pettiness and avarice. In the background operated a highly developed organisation of Public Health, whose action however was frustrated by the medical ignorance and the economic poverty of a pre-industrial society.'

34. Post, *op. cit.*, 36. There are of course many studies in this area – for another recent paper, see A.B. Appleby, 'Nutrition and disease: the case of London 1550-1750', *Journal of Interdisciplinary History, 6*, 1975-6, 1-22. Appleby suggests that environmental factors appear to have been less important than one might expect in the case of London mortality. Largely independent of environmental factors, the course of disease may have to be treated as an autonomous influence on population growth.
35. D.V. Glass and D.E.C. Eversley (eds.), *Population in History*, London, 1965; E.A. Wrigley (ed.), *Introduction to English Historical Demography*, London, 1966, and his *Population and History*, London, 1969; T.H. Hollingsworth, *Historical Demography*, London, 1969, and R.S. Schofield, 'Historical demography: some possibilities and some limitations', *Transactions of the Royal Historical Society, 21*, 1971, 119-32.
36. M.C. Buer, *Health, Wealth and Population in the Early Days of the Industrial Revolution*, London, 1926; and G. Talbot Griffith, *Population Problems of the Age of Malthus*, Cambridge, 1926.
37. T. McKeown and R.G. Brown, 'Medical evidence related to English population changes in the eighteenth century', *Population Studies, 9*, 1955-6, 285-307.
38. P.E. Razzell, 'Population change in eighteenth century England: a reinterpretation', *Economic History Review, 18*, 1965, 312-32; E.M. Sigsworth, 'Gateways to death? Medicine, hospitals and mortality, 1700-1850', in P. Mathias (ed.), *Science and Society 1600-1900*, Cambridge, 1972, and Woodward, *op. cit.*
39. D.E.C. Eversley, 'A survey of population in an area of Worcestershire from 1660 to 1850', *Population Studies, 10*, 1956-7, 230-53, and J.D. Chambers, *Population, Economy and Society in Pre-industrial England*, London, 1972. There are innumerable papers and books relating to these aspects of population change. For an excellent summary and assessment see Peter Mathias, 'Disease, medicine and demography in Britain during the industrial revolution', *Annales Cisalpines d'Histoire Sociale*, Serie 1-No. 4, 1973, 145-84.
40. For a typical example of the new approach see E.A. Wrigley, 'Mortality in pre-industrial England: the example of Colyton, Devon over three centuries', *Daedalus, 97*, 1968, 546-80. A wider ranging survey can be found in Peter Laslett, *The World We Have Lost*, 2nd edn., London, 1971 – especially chap. five.
41. M.J. Cullen, *The Statistical Movement in Early Victorian Britain – the Foundations of Empirical Social Research*, Hassocks and New York, 1975.
42. *Ibid.*, p. 149.
43. Samuel P. Hays, 'Historical social research. Concept, method and technique', *Journal of Interdisciplinary History, 4*, 1974-5, 475-81.
44. *Ibid.*, 481.
45. For a classic account using such techniques see E.P. Thompson, *The*

Making of the English Working Class, London, 1963 and 1968.

46. Bruch Mazlish, 'What is psychohistory?', *Transactions of the Royal Historical Society, 21,* 1971, 79-99; Robert J. Lifton (ed.), *Explorations in Psychohistory,* New York, 1974; J. Barzun, *Clio and the Doctors: Psychohistory, Quanto-history and History,* Chicago, 1974; and Fred Weinstein and Gerald M. Platt, 'The coming crisis in psychohistory', *Journal of Modern History, 47,* 1975, 202-28.
47. D.R. Allen, 'Florence Nightingale: towards a psychohistorical interpretation', *Journal of Interdisciplinary History, 6,* 1975-6, 23-45.
48. Oliver MacDonagh, 'The nineteenth century revolution in government: a reappraisal', *Historical Journal,* 1, 1958, 52-67. See also J.B. Brebner, 'Laissez-faire and state intervention in nineteenth century Britain, *Journal of Economic History, 8* (supplement), 1948, 59-73. For the debate following MacDonagh's thesis see Henry Parris, 'The nineteenth century revolution in government: a reappraisal reappraised', *Historical Journal, 3,* 1960, 17-37; Jennifer Hart, 'Nineteenth-century social reform: a tory interpretation of history', *Past and Present,* no. 31, 1965, 39-61; Valerie Cromwell, 'Interpretations of nineteenth century administration: an analysis', *Victorian Studies, 9,* 1965-6, 245-55, and Gillian Sutherland, 'Recent trends in administrative history', *Victorian Studies, 13,* 1969-70, 408-11. For a summary of the arguments for and against MacDonagh's thesis see Arthur J. Taylor, *Laissez-faire and State Intervention in Nineteenth Century Britain,* London, 1972; and Gillian Sutherland (ed.), *Studies in the Growth of Nineteenth Century Government,* London, 1972. For a detailed study of the early Victorian period see W.C. Lubenow, *The Politics of Government Growth, Early Victorian Attitudes Toward State Intervention, 1833-1848,* Newton Abbot, 1971.
49. Steven J. Novak 'Professionalism and bureaucracy: English doctors and the Victorian public health administration', *Journal of Social History, 6,* 1972-3, 440-62. Novak argues that if the impact of the civil service on the medical profession was disappointing, the force of professionalism was a major factor in shaping the public health bureaucracy.
50. Derek Fraser, *The Evolution of the British Welfare State – A History of Social Policy Since the Industrial Revolution,* London 1973, p. 71.
51. *Ibid.,* p.114.
52. For a full account see Frank Honigsbaum, *The Struggle for the Ministry of Health,* Occasional Papers in Social Administration, no. 37, London, 1970.
53. Ruth G. Hodgkinson, *The Origins of the National Health Service. The Medical Services of the New Poor Law 1834-1871,* London, 1967; Jeanne L. Brand, *Doctors and the State: the British Medical Profession and Government Action in Public Health 1870-1912,* Baltimore, 1965, and Rosemary Stevens, *Medical Practice in Modern England. The Impact of Specialisation and State Medicine,* New Haven and London, 1966. For a comparative analysis see Rosemary Stevens, *American Medicine and Public Interest,* New Haven and London, 1971.
54. Bentley B. Gilbert, *The Evolution of National Insurance in Great Britain: The Origins of the Welfare State,* London, 1966, and his *British Social Policy 1914-1939,* London, 1970.
55. On the Poor Law, amongst many others see Michael E. Rose, *The English Poor Law 1780-1930,* Newton Abbot, 1971, and his *The Relief of Poverty 1834-1914,* London 1972. For a study which combines the use of local history see E.C. Midwinter, *Social Administration in Lancashire, 1820-1860,* Manchester, 1968. On the National Health Service, again from

amongst a plethora of published material, see H. Eckstein, *The English Health Service*, Cambridge, Mass., 1959; A Lindsey, *Socialised Medicine in England and Wales: the National Health Service 1948-1961*, London, 1962, and A.J. Willcocks, *The Creation of the National Health Service*, London, 1967. For a study of mental health services see Kathleen Jones, *A History of the Mental Health Services*, London, 1972.

56. On this see Maurice Wright, *Treasury Control of the Civil Service 1854-1874*, Oxford, 1969, and his 'Treasury Control 1854-1914', in Sutherland, *op. cit.*, pp. 195-226; Roy M. MacLeod, *Treasury Control and Social Administration: A Study of Establishment Growth at the Local Government Board 1871-1905*, Occasional papers on Social Administration, no. 23, London, 1968, and his 'The frustration of state medicine 1880-1899', *Medical History*, *11*, 1967, 15-40.
57. Rene Dubos, *The Mirage of Health: Utopias, Progress and Biological Change*, New York, 1959, p. 22.
58. *Ibid.* For a complete discussion of this point see R. Campbell, 'Economics and health in the history of ideas', *Annales Cisalpines d'Histoire Sociale*, Serie 1 – No. 4, 1973, 63-82.
59. Keith Thomas, *Religion and Decline of Magic. Studies in Popular Beliefs in Sixteenth and Seventeenth Century England*, London, 1971. See also Alan Macfarlane's parallel study, *Witchcraft in Tudor and Stuart England. A Regional and Comparative Study*, London, 1970.
60. Thomas, *op. cit.*, p. 178.
61. *Ibid.*
62. *Ibid.*, p. 210
63. Henry Miller, 'The literature of medicine', *Times Literary Supplement*, 29 March 1974, 316.
64. Henry E. Sigerist, 'The Social History of Medicine', *Western Journal of Obstetrics and Gynecology*, *48*, 1940, 714.
65. See for example T.S. Kuhn, *The Structure of Scientific Revolutions*, 2nd edn., Chicago, 1970
66. For the composition of one of these see Roy M. MacLeod, 'The X Club: a scientific network in late-Victorian England', *Notes and Records of the Royal Society*, *24*, 1969-70, 305-22, and J. Vernon Jensen, 'The X Club: fraternity of British scientists', *British Journal for the History of Science*, *5*, 1970-1, 63-72. See also M.B. Hall, 'The Royal Society's role in diffusion of information in the seventeenth century', *Notes and Records of the Royal Society*, *29*, 1975, 173-92.
67. Charles Creighton, *A History of Epidemics in Britain*, London, 1891 (vol. 1) and 1894 (vol. II). In this context and as an example in this genre see Daphne A. Roe, *A Plague of Corn. The Social History of Pellagra*, Ithaca and London, 1973.
68. Barbara Rodgers, 'The Social Science Association, 1957-1886', *Manchester School*, *20*, 1952, 283-310; Michael Millman 'The influence of the Social Science Association on hospital planning in Victorian England', *Medical History*, *18*, 1974, 122-37; B. Hill, 'Statistical result of the Contagious Diseases Acts', *Journal of the Royal Statistical Society*, *33*, 1870, 463-85; F.B. Smith, 'Ethics and Disease in the later nineteenth century: the Contagious Diseases Acts', *Historical Studies*, *15*, 1971, 118-35; D. and J. Walkowitz, 'We are not beasts of the field: prostitution and the poor in Plymouth and Southampton under the Contagious Diseases Acts', *Feminist Studies*, *1*, 1973, 73-106; Ann Beck, 'Issues in the anti-vaccination movement in England', *Medical History*, *4*, 1960, 310-21, and Roy M. MacLeod, 'Law, medicine and public opinion: the resistance to

compulsory health legislation, 1870-1907', *Public Law*, 1967, 107-28 and 189-211. For a general comment see O.R. McGregor, 'Social research and social policy in the nineteenth century', *British Journal of Sociology, 8*, 1957, 146-57. On Victorian prostitution and venereal disease see *Prostitution in the Victorian Age*, with an introduction by Keith Nield, Farnborough, 1973; and E.M. Sigsworth and T.J. Wyke, 'A study of Victorian prostitution and venereal disease', in Martha Vicinus (ed.), *Suffer and Be Still*, Bloomington and London, 1972, pp. 77-99 and 216-22.

69. The majority of the references cited in this paper have been from the literature written in English. For a review of continental studies see A.E. Imhof and O. Larsen, *Sozialgeschichte und Medizin*, Oslo and Stuttgart, 1975.
70. H.J. Perkin, 'Social history', in H.P.R. Finberg (ed.), *Approaches to History*, London, 1962, p. 59.
71. George Rosen, *From Medical Police to Social Medicine. Essays on the History of Health Care*, New York, 1974, p. 2.
72. Ruth G. Hodgkinson, 'The social environment of British medical service and practice in the nineteenth century', in William C. Gibson (ed.), *British Contributions to Medical Science*, London, 1971, p. 45.
73. Ida Macalpine and Richard Hunter, ' The Pathography of the past', *Times Literary Supplement*, 15 March 1974, 256.
74. George Rosen, 'Health, history and the social sciences', *Social Science and Medicine, 7*, 1973, 236
75. Sigerist (1936), *op. cit.*, 6.
76. *Ibid.*, 5.
77. Malcolm Johnson (ed.), *Medical Sociology in Britain – a Register of Research and Teaching*, Leeds, 1974. In this see in particular David Richards' light-hearted but sympathetic review of the predominant trends, 'The Medical Sociology Group: 1969-1974', pp. xi-xiv.
78. Holloway, *op. cit.*
79. Wilson, *op. cit.*, 103.
80. S.W.F. Holloway, 'The Apothecaries Act, 1815: a reinterpretation', *Medical History, 10*, 1966, 107-29, and 221-35.
81. S.W.F. Holloway, 'Medical education in England 1830-1858: a sociological analysis', *History, 49*, 1964, 299.
82. Ivan Waddington, 'The struggle to reform the Royal College of Physicians 1767-1771' – a sociological analysis, *Medical History, 17*, 1973, 107-26, and his 'The development of medical ethics – a sociological analysis', *Medical History, 19*, 1975, 36-51.
83. Ivan Waddington, 'The role of the hospital in the development of modern medicine: a sociological analysis', *Sociology, 7*, 1973, 211-24.
84. N.D. Jewson, 'Medical knowledge and the patronage system in eighteenth century England', *Sociology, 8*, 1974, 369-85.
85. On nursing see Brian Abel-Smith, *A History of the Nursing Profession*, London, 1960. For studies of the development of dentistry see N. David Richards, 'Dentistry in England in the 1840s: the first indications of a movement towards professionalisation', *Medical History, 12*, 1968, 137-52; his 'The dental profession', in F.N.L. Poynter (ed.), *Medicine and Science in the 1860s*, London, 1968, pp. 267-88; and his 'Dentistry a hundred years ago: Charles James Fox – the forgotten man', *British Dental Journal, 132*, 1972, 235-42. For a wider review of the development and status of dentistry see also his 'Dentistry in Great Britain – some sociologic perspectives', *Milbank Memorial Fund Quarterly, 49*, 1971 (3, part 2), 133-69. On midwifery see Jean E. Donnison, *The Development of the*

Profession of Midwife in England 1750-1902, PhD thesis, University of London, 1974, and her forthcoming, *Midwives and Medical Men,* London, 1977.

86. N. David Richards and Arthur J. Willcocks, 'The level of dental health: the field for study', in Gordon McLachlan (ed.), *Problems and Progress in Medical Care. Essays on Current Research,* second series, London, 1966. pp. 313-38, and J.S. Bulman, N.D. Richards, G.L. Slack and A.J. Willcocks, *Demand and Need for Dental Care: A socio-Dental Survey,* London, 1968.
87. Eliot Freidson, 'Client control and medical practice', *American Journal of Sociology, 65,* 1959-60, 374-82: his *Patients' Views of Medical Practice,* New York, 1961; and his *Professional Dominance: the Social Structure of Medical Care,* Chicago, 1970.
88. For a general introduction to this area see David Mechanic, *Medical Sociology, A Selective Review,* New York, 1968; and R.M. Coe, *Sociology of Medicine,* New York, 1970. See also E.G. Jaco (ed.), *Patients, Physicians and Illness,* New York, 1958; Howard E. Freeman, Sol Levine and Leo G. Reeder (eds.), *Handbook of Medical Sociology,* Englewood Cliffs, New Jersey, 1963; and W. Richard Scott and Edmund H. Volkart (eds.), *Medical Care – Readings in the Sociology of Medical Institutions,* New York and London, 1966.
89. See for example David Robinson, *Patients, Practitioners and Medical Care: Aspects of Medical Sociology,* London, 1973; Caroline Cox and Adrianne Mead (eds.), *A Sociology of Medical Practice,* London, 1975, and David Tuckett (ed.), *An Introduction to Medical Sociology,* London, 1976.
90. For a further clarification of this distinction see Robert Straus, 'The nature and status of medical sociology', *American Sociological Review, 22,* 1957, 200-4, and Margot Jefferys, 'Sociology and medicine: separation or symbiosis', *Lancet,* 1969, *i,* 1111-16. For a recent critique on the present state of medical sociology see Freidson (1970), *op. cit.,* pp. 41-58.
91. R.M. Titmuss, *Social Policy – An Introduction,* London, 1974, p. 16.
92. *Ibid.,* p. 15.
93. H.E. Sigerist, ' The special position of the sick', in M.I. Roemer (ed.), *H.E. Sigerist on the Sociology of Medicine,* New York, 1960, chap. 2; L.J. Henderson, 'Physician and patient as a social system', *New England Journal of Medicine, 212,* 1935, 819-23, and T. Parsons, *The Social System,* London, 1951.
94. David Mechanic, 'The concept of illness behaviour', *Journal of Chronic Diseases, 15,* 1962, 189-94. See also his *op. cit.,* pp. 115-57
95. David Mechanic, 'Illness and social disability: some problems in analysis', *Pacific Sociological Review, 2,* 1959, 37-41.
96. E.L. Koos, *The Health of Regionville: What People Thought and Did About it,* New York, 1954.
97. For development of this theme see Andrew C. Twaddle, 'Illness and deviance', *Social Science and Medicine, 7,* 1973, 751-62, and his 'The concept of health status', *Social Science and Medicine, 8,* 1974, 29-38.
98. Mechanic (1968), *op. cit.,* pp. 130-1, and 142-55.
99. For studies of the way people use medicines and deal with symptoms with and without a doctor's help see M.E.J. Wadsworth, W.J.H. Butterfield and R. Blaney, *Health and Sickness: The Choice of Treatment,* London, 1971, and Karen Dunnel and Ann Cartwright, *Medicine Takers, Prescribers and Hoarders,* London, 1972.
100. For a recent and comprehensive review of the literature on use of health services see John B. McKinlay, 'Some approaches and problems in the study of the use of services – an overview', *Journal of Health and Social*

Behaviour, 13, 1972, 115-52. See also J.G. Anderson, 'Health services utilisation: framework and review', *Health Services Research 8,* 1973, 184-99.
101. On this see respectively E.A. Suchman, 'Stages of illness and medical care, *Journal of Health and Human Behaviour, 6,* 1965, 114-28; I.K. Zola, 'Pathways to the doctor – from person to patient', *Social Science and Medicine, 7,* 1973, 677-89; and E.A. Suchman, 'Social patterns of illness and medical care', *Journal of Health and Human Behaviour, 6,* 1965, 2-16; his 'Health orientations and medical care', *American Journal of Public Health, 56,* 1966, 97-104, and his 'Social factors in illness behaviour' *Milbank Memorial Fund Quarterly, 47,* (1, Part 1), 1969, 85-93.
102. Freidson (1959-60), *op. cit.*
103. Holloway (1964), *op. cit.,* 318.
104. On this see in particular Freidson (1961), *op. cit.* and Mechanic (1968), *op. cit.,* pp. 158-91. For a useful review of this field see also John D. Stoeckle, Irving K. Zola and Gerald E. Davidson, 'On going to see the doctor, the contributions of the patient to the decision to seek medical aid', *Journal of Chronic Diseases, 16,* 1963, 975-89. For a recent study of patients' attitudes to their general practitioners see Ann Cartwright, *Patients and Their Doctors, A Study of General Practice,* London, 1967.
105. Leo G. Reeder, 'The patient-client as a consumer: some observations of the changing professional-client relationship', *Journal of Health and Social Behaviour, 13,* 1972, 406-12.
106. Gerry Stimson and Barbara Webb, *Going to See the Doctor: the Consultation Process in General Practice,* London, 1975.
107 See for example Thomas S. Szasz and Marc H. Hollender, 'A contribution to the philosophy of medicine. The basic models of the doctor-patient relationship', *Archives of General Medicine, 97,* 1956, 585-92; Samuel W. Bloom, *The Doctor and his Patient. A Sociological Interpretation,* New York, 1963, and Robert N. Wilson, 'Patient-practitioner relationships', in Freeman, Levine and Reeder, *op. cit.,* pp. 273-95.
108. Eliot Freidson, *Profession of Medicine. A Study of the Sociology of Applied Knowledge,* New York, 1970 (b), pp. 317-18.
109. Marshall H. Becker and Lois A. Maiman, 'Sociobehavioural determinants of compliance with health and medical care recommendations', *Medical Care, 13,* 1975, 10-24.
110. A voluminous literature in this field may be cited, but see especially B. Barber, 'Some problems in the sociology of professions', *Daedalus, 92,* 1963, 669-88; A.M. Carr-Saunders and P.A. Wilson, *The Professions,* Oxford, 1933; Freidson (1970 b), *op. cit.;* E.C. Hughes, 'Professions', *Daedalus, 92,* 1963, 655-68; J.A. Jackson (ed.), *Professions and Professionalization,* Cambridge, 1970; T.J. Johnson, *Professions and Power,* London, 1972; G.L. Millerson, *The Qualifying Associations,* London, 1964; W.J. Reader, *Professional Men,* London, 1966, and H.M. Vollmer and D.L. Mills (eds.), *Professionalization,* Englewood Cliffs, New Jersey, 1966.
111. Freidson (1970), *op. cit.,* p. 3.
112. *Ibid.*
113. Eliot Freidson (ed.), *The Hospital in Modern Society,* New York, 1963. For a study of patients' reactions to hospital see Ann Cartwright, *Human Relations and Hospital Care,* London, 1964.
114. J.S. Coleman, E. Katz and H. Menzel, *Medical Innovation – A Diffusion Study,* Indianapolis, 1966. See also E. Katz, 'Social itinerary of technical change: two studies of the diffusion of innovation', *Human Organisation, 20,* 1961, 70-87.
115. E.S. Rogers, *Diffusion of Innovations,* New York, 1962, and A.E. Niehoff

(ed.), *A Casebook of Social Change*, Chicago, 1966.

116. Edmund D. Pellegrino, 'Medicine, history and the idea of man', *Annals of the American Academy of Political and Social Science, 346*, 1963, 10. See also Henry E. Sigerist, *A History of Medicine*, vol.I, New York, 1951, p. 31.
117. Charles Webster, *The Great Instauration*, London, 1975.
118. On this see Steven Polgar, 'Health and human behaviour: areas of interest common to the social and medical sciences', *Current Anthropology, 3*, 1962, 159-205, and his 'Health action in cross-cultural perspective' in Freeman, Levine and Reeder, *op. cit.*, pp. 397-419. For a general introduction to this subject area see also Iago Galdston (ed.), *Medicine and Anthropology*, New York, 1959; Margaret Read, *Culture, Health and Disease*, London, 1966, and F.N.L. Poynter (ed.), *Medicine and Culture*, London, 1969. For a recent attempt to synthesise the various social scientific and medical approaches see Horacio Fabrega, *Disease and Social Behaviour: An Interdisciplinary Perspective*, London, 1974.
119. For an introduction to studies of technological change see E.H. Spicer, *Human Problems in Technological Change*, New York, 1952; Margaret Mead (ed.), *Cultural Patterns and Technical Change* Paris, 1953; Benjamin D. Paul (ed.), *Health, Culture and Community*, New York, 1955; G.M. Foster, *Traditional Cultures and the Impact of Technological Change*, New York, 1962; W.H. Goodenough, *Co-operation in Change*, New York, 1963, and Niehoff, *op. cit.*
120. On the implications of this point in relation to the development of health education see N. David Richards, 'Methods and effectiveness of health education: the past, present and future of social scientific involvement', *Social Science and Medicine, 9*, 1975, 141-56, and his 'Towards a redefinition of health education: the role of the social sciences', *Community Health, 7*, 1976, 135-43.
121. In addition to Macfarlane, *op. cit.*, and Thomas, *op. cit.*, see also G. Zilboorg, *The Medical Man and the Witch During the Renaissance*, New York, 1935, and E.H. Ackerknecht, 'Natural diseases and rational treatment in primitive medicine', *Bulletin of the History of Medicine, 19*, 1946, 467-97. Two recent anthropoligical studies of witchraft are M. Douglas (ed.), *Witchcraft: Confessions and Accusations*, London, 1970, and M. Marwick (ed.), *Witchcraft and Sorcery: Selected Readings*, Harmondsworth, 1972.
122. Monica Wilson, 'Witch beliefs and social structure', *American Journal of Sociology, 56*, 1950-1,313.
123. On insanity see for example George Rosen, *Madness in Society: Chapters in the Historical Sociology of Mental Illness*, London, 1968. Note also his comment that 'along a spectrum of human behaviour ranging from that considered normal to that regarded as abnormal, there is some point at which a judgment is made and an individual is designated as mad. In practice, the dividing line between normality and abnormality, between sanity and insanity, is not always easily established.' (Rosen (1973), *Social Science and Medicine*, 235.) For the development of mental health services in Britain see Jones, *op. cit.*, who, however, says very little about patients, where they came from, what was wrong with them, and who, if anyone, treated them. For a history of institutions for the insane in England, see William L. Parry-Jones, *The Trade in Lunacy: A Study in Private Madhouses in England in the Eighteenth and Nineteenth Centuries*, London, 1972. Important, too, will be an understanding of the iconography of mental disease.

124. George Rosen, 'People, disease and emotion: some new problems for research in medical history', *Bulletin of the History of Medicine, 41*, 1967, 20. For recent developments in the fields of historical and social geography see E.W. Gilbert, 'Pioneer maps of health and disease in England', *Geographical Journal, 124*, 1958, 172-83; E.M. Rawstron and B.E. Coates, *Regional Variations in Britain*, London, 1971, and G. Melvyn Howe, *Man, Environment and Disease in Britain*, Newton Abbot, 1972.
125. W. Pagel, 'Henry Sigerist', *Medical History, 1*, 1957, 286.
126. F.N.L. Poynter, 'Medicine and the historians', *Bulletin of the History of Medicine, 30*, 1956, 429.
127. D. Guthrie, 'Whither medical history?', *Medical History, 1*, 1957, 309.
128. J.F. Hutchinson, 'Historical method and the social history of medicine', *Medical History, 17*, 1973, 423.
129. *Ibid.*, 427
130. L.S. King, 'An interdisciplinary approach to medical history', *Clio Medica, 9*, 1974, 6.
131. Thomas McKeown, 'A sociological approach to the history of medicine', *Medical History, 14*, 1970, 342 – reprinted in modified form in Gordon McLachlan and Thomas McKeown (eds.), *Medical History and Medical Care – A Symposium of Perspectives*, London, 1971.
132. Ivan Illich, *Medical Nemesis, The Expropriation of Health*, London, 1975, p.87.
133. Freidson (1970), *op. cit.*
134. Illich, *op. cit.*, p. 92.
135. Rosen (1973, *Social Science and Medicine*), 238-9.

2 POPULAR THEORIES OF GENERATION: THE EVOLUTION OF ARISTOTLE'S WORKS, THE STUDY OF AN ANACHRONISM

Janet Blackman

Keith Thomas,[1] and other authors such as Alan Macfarlane,[2] have begun to look at the role played in this country in past time by various magical rites, witchcraft, folklore, superstitions, and the way these were rooted out, absorbed into, and replaced by organised religion, with its alternative explanations of the universe, source of life, good versus evil, health versus disease, etc. This is a fascinating story analysing an aspect of the transition from Western medieval thought and culture, and its dependence on the ancient world, to concepts more appropriate to the modern age and the emergent nation state. Part of that transition involved the discovery, understanding and acceptance of new scientific ideas which struck at the heart not only of laws, such as those of motion, as they were then understood, but also at concepts of matter, like the generation of life and the functions of the body, which to then had dominated science and medicine through Arabic, Greek and Latin sources.

How were such new ideas absorbed, reinterpreted or even rejected at the popular level? There must have been an on-going understanding, largely oral, handed down from generation to generation, explaining natural phenomena, bodily functions and malfunctions. This was probably derived from a conglomeration of ideas, linked together in some way, and this too may have adjusted to the new notions; but how, why and over what time-span?

There has recently been renewed interest among historians in the scientific revolution of the sixteenth and seventeenth centuries attempting to discover what might be called the sociological origins of this scientific renaissance.[3] Christopher Hill has suggested that the rise of new scientific ideas formed part of the shift by which urban and industrial values replaced those more appropriate to an agrarian society.[4] Others have seen a greater division between the growth of technical expertise associated with industrialisation and the development of scientific ideas. Rabb has pointed in a footnote to the 'essential differences between the artisan's utilitarian aims and the scientist's conceptual aims'.[5] The other dimension of the scientific revolution of which we know and understand even less is that of popular ideas about science and scientific concepts, how they emerged and were circulated and the nature of their social significance.

Kuhn, in his studies of scientific revolutions, has been concerned with the professional scientist and scientific knowledge in the purist or intellectual sense.[6] At the same time what he has said in his re-assessment of the nature of scientific revolutions is of interest in attempting to define and understand the growth of a popular form of science. How did popular 'scientific' explanations of natural phenomena evolve? They used presumably some intellectual base – from which they developed over the centuries, often by word of mouth – in the form of ideas, folklore, theories handed down from generation to generation which served a number of purposes. At the same time there may have been some links with developments in intellectual or professional scientific understanding. Kuhn noted that in the professional scientific revolutions there appeared to be a historical process whereby some discoveries and beliefs are deemed by a later age to have led to advances in scientific knowledge, whereas others, despite their integral role in the past system of knowledge, are regarded as not having this merit and have become myths in a later age.[7] The evolution of popular science may be subject to the same process as it develops its own body of knowledge and literature in tracts and treatises as well as an oral tradition. But there is also the question of the links, if any, and over what time-scale, between this popular form and the professional. There may be factors within a society which help to determine the development of popular concepts of scientific principles whereby they are assimilated into general knowledge and literature for the enlightenment of the non-scientist, a process which may have its own historical time-scale. This, in turn may or may not be closely related to that of intellectual advances in knowledge. For instance, the popular jettisoning of ideas already regarded, even condemned, as myths or out of date by scientists,[8] is probably a slower process, especially where the new professional concepts involve a different system or logic of analysis from that of the popular.

The acceptance and integration into existing popular ideas of new data and principles is a difficult process for the historian to identify and explain. Why should it happen? Where would the pressure come from and how would it be exerted? The distinction between lay and professional was more blurred until recent time. At the same time this process of assimilation of new principles at the popular everyday level involves a measure of social acceptance of these ideas and in a form which may not entirely overthrow the existing popular ideas and beliefs. Paradoxically the effect of this may be to give the popular forms of knowledge a potency which far outlasts their intellectual validity. The transition from Aristotelian to non-Aristotelian ideas may be a particularly dramatic example of this process. The battles at the intellectual level between the different schools of thought may have their own history, but how did the ordinary man or woman find out about revolutions in the understanding of matter, origins of life, etc.? Can we envisage a popular system of knowledge which relates somehow to the intellectual? There may be some kind of relationship, both sympathetic and oppositional, between the popular and the intellectual at a particular period. As the latter changes, this relationship continues in some way between the new system of knowledge as it emerges at both intellectual and popular levels.

The tension in a period of change between intellectual advances in knowledge and popular understanding, and acceptance of them must have involved much more than a time-lag. An elucidation of this point will be attempted in this essay by looking at medical knowledge at the scientific and professional level and at popular ideas on generation. Here the distinction is clearer between the professional and the lay – in the sense of the popular. There may, however, also be strata of lay understanding ranging, for instance, from the educated to the ill-informed. Enough popular Aristotelian literature, especially medical tracts, has survived in various forms from the sixteenth century in Europe to give us some insight into this.

Thomas has observed that the invention of printing made possible 'the preservation and dissemination of many different systems of thought, deriving from other societies and sometimes dating from the remote classical past', which present the historian with 'so many different layers of belief and levels in sophistication'.[9]

One of the most important forms of popular quasi-scientific publication, not only in Britain and Western Europe but also exported to North America, has been 'medical', offering the layman and, in particular, the woman advice on a variety of physical and personal characteristics, and correctives for their malfunction. Included also in the popularisation process were sexual relations and childbirth, which remained for centuries uneasily on the fringe of medicine because it was preoccupied, or appeared to be preoccupied, only with the diseased body. The manuals printed for the woman's assistance drew on a variety of sources: the housewife's commonsense observations and inherited knowledge of medical remedies were intermixed with information and ideas from ancient herbals, systems of divination such as physiognomy, and a multitude of translations from the Greek, Arabic and Latin of classical texts, and their imitators. Of particular interest in this popular literature on scientific and medical topics are the collections of problems in question and answer form, originally compiled in the fourteenth and fifteenth centuries, which draw on earlier collections such as the ancient Salernitan Questions.[10]

One of the most popular of these problem books was usually attributed to Aristotle and eventually formed part of the compilation known as *Aristotle's Works.* This compendium of medical or quasi-medical knowledge was issued over many centuries in numerous editions. Sometimes a new edition incorporated new ideas and interpretations, and it may be possible to define, however indistinctly, through this particular publication, a process of assimilation of more modern concepts into what must have become a patchwork of information and advice. *Aristotle's Works,* and that section of it entitled *Aristotle's Masterpiece,* have been well-known sex handbooks for over three hundred years. Until attacked by some members of the medical profession in the 1930s and earlier, the compilation had long been possibly the most popular source of information on sexual relations and childbirth – subjects which ensured that it remained an obscure and undercover publication, regarded socially as being of doubtful taste, yet much read and consulted by both men and women. It went through numerous editions and revisions in the seventeenth and eighteenth centuries, and possibly earlier, and became a late-Victorian bestseller amongst that kind of literature.

Aristotle's Works and the *Masterpiece* are still published as popular tracts on the origins of life, conception, pregnancy, childbirth, signs of the zodiac, etc. – very much like an almanac or collection of folklore – in which the ordinary man and woman may find useful and titillating information on the 'facts of life'. There appears even today to be a common but almost latent or unstated knowledge of this publication. It is popular in the sense that it is widely known, not always in great detail, rarely mentioned, yet circulated as a midly pornographic piece of literature about matters which until very recently were seldom openly discussed.[11]

It is probable that the continuing publication of this work is very much the last remnant of a much stronger popular demand and usage that began to grow at the end of the nineteenth century. An increasingly literate population, with the assistance in many editions of diagrams and pictures, began to read and pass on the sort of literature that had been available to a smaller readership centuries before. Michael Sadleir (M.T.H. Sadler), in his historical novel of London's underworld and underprivileged, set in the latter part of the nineteenth century –

Forlorn Sunset – chose 'The Genuine Editions of ARISTOTLE, the Famous Philosopher' as an example of the literature of doubtful propriety available from low-class booksellers of that period.[12] A publication such as this, known for centuries in various editions, probably acquired therefore a new popularity, a much extended readership, by trading in part both on its medical-style information, and on its prurient reputation. A bookseller's advertisement of 1903 for this kind of literature shows very clearly this juxtaposition. John Simpson Symington of Leeds gave a list of his stock on the back of the thirty-sixth edition of Dr H.A. Allbutt's then norotious medical guide. *Aristotle's Masterpiece* he listed immediately below Allbutt's *The Wife's Handbook* (first published in 1886), and priced it at one shilling (5p).

Joseph Needham has suggested that such publications 'reprinted and modified a hundred-fold, formed and still form to-day, the main source of instruction on sexual and embryological matters for the working-class populations of Western Europe', and referred particularly to *Aristotle's Works* as an example.[13] A.L. Rowse has borne testimony to this in his autobiography, where he comments on his writing home from university as an undergraduate:

> From this November dates the first of the letters home that my mother took to keeping; pretty simple they had to be; my parents didn't find it easy to read handwriting. This one is mostly about my Labour Club activities – no use confiding to them my troubles with Tait and Tout, Rousseau and Aristotle. (Aristotle would have meant to my mother, as secretly to Victorian women, his book on child-bearing: unmentionable. But I knew that book was secreted in her chest of drawers in the old home. That was what the sage meant to the people).[14]

Peck has made the same point in a footnote to his English translation of Aristotle's *Generation of Animals:* 'Among the less learned . . . the outstanding achievement of Aristotle in this branch of study has been for at least the last three centuries acknowledged by the title of the popular handbook known as *Aristotle's Masterpiece*'.[15]

The popularity for many centuries of *Aristotle's Works,* or that section of it called *Aristotle's Masterpiece,* can be explained at least in part by the nature of its contents. The popular manuals produced for women on domestic economy, in the nineteenth century especially, were more concerned with giving advice on roles to be played and standards of social behaviour to be attained by them as wives and mothers. The works of Mrs Ellis are probably the most well-known nineteenth-century examples, especially her *Women of England, and their Social Duties, and Domestic Habits,* and her *Daughters of England.*[16] Powell has analysed the same type of publication in earlier centuries.[17] Authors like these gave some advice of a practical nature on the feeding and bathing of a baby, the choosing of a wet nurse, etc., but there was no advice on intercourse, conception, pregnancy and the delivery of the baby. Their comments began with the moment the new child first drew breath with not a hint of what had gone before.[18] Mrs Sarah Hale, for instance, in her *New Household Receipt-Book* opens her section on children with the words: 'Immediately on the birth of the child, it should be received into soft fine flannel.'[19] Another form of popular literature, such as Buchan's *Domestic Medicine*[20] with its more precise medical purpose, was concerned with diseases, their prevention and cure, 'shewing people what is in their own power',[21] and so was of little guidance to women on natural processes such as pregnancy and childbirth, which receive only a brief mention.[22] None of these publications were of much assistance to young women and men beginning to seek knowledge about sexual relations, or for the newly married woman expecting her first child. It is not surprising, therefore, that *Aristotle's Works,* often illustrated with anatomical diagrams in later editions, and with the technical or gynaecological information which could be extracted from its other contents, maintained its popularity for so long. Yet to modern eyes this is a curious book, dealing with pregnancy, childbirth and related topics in terms which would be regarded now as ancient myths. It could be dismissed as worthless, a sort of titillating chapbook; on the other hand it has been for a very long time the only kind of popular medical and natural science handbook which was available to the layman and woman who possessed little knowledge of such matters other than their own experiences and the tales of others.

How it was used and how the information it contained was accepted, understood, interpreted and practised can only be guessed at. Another question is why, when by the end of the nineteenth century more medically reliable, modern guides were beginning to be printed in Britain and also imported from America in some quantity, it continued to circulate. There are nonetheless all sorts of clues as to why such a publication remained in some sense 'useful', even though in medical and scientific terms it was largely anachronistic and Aristotelian in concept, and its medical explanations were based on humoral pathology. It is therefore perhaps more appropriate to ask in what sense was *Aristotle's Works* anachronistic and to whom? It may have been acceptable and much referred to because of its longevity, a source of information well-known as a basic text handed down from generation to generation, by women perhaps more than men. Sometimes separate sections were printed as handouts and tracts which were sold at fairs and markets, while leather-bound copies graced the bookcases and dressing-tables of the more well-to-do. It may not be an exaggeration, therefore, to suggest that this is an enormously important piece of documentation, an example of the type of popular literature quite widely available from which ideas and systems of thought or particular linkages between certain phenomena and events were formed and came to be accepted by the layman. The main topics covered were medical, dealing with bodily functions, especially female, their disorders and treatments. It also had a social significance, influencing perceptions of such matters. Its anachronism lay in its long history as a popular pseudo-scientific tract, separate to a large extent, but yet not entirely so, from the advances being made in scientific and medical knowledge. It is that long life, the continuation of an Aristotelian system of ideas at the popular level until recently which needs explaining as well as the impact made by such ideas. There may have been links with professional science, but this again could not have been a simple matter of assimilation of new ideas by editorial additions and revisions, but must have involved some degree of social acceptability at the lay level, or at least an assessment by the editor of its acceptability. How was this achieved?

The survival and use of *Aristotle's Works* over several centuries in Britain, Western Europe and finally North America may offer an opportunity of looking closely at a particular publication. The four editions that have been studied here in some detail date from the late seventeenth, the late eighteenth, the mid-nineteenth and the early twentieth centuries. No assessment has been made as to how far this publication was representative of its genre at any of these dates, although reference will be made to other popular works on midwifery, female disorders, etc. etc.

What sort of publication was *Aristotle's Works*? The nineteenth-century edition used in this analysis is called *Aristotle's Works containing The Masterpiece, Directions for Midwives and Counsel and Advice to Child-Bearing Women; with various useful remedies,* and was printed by The Booksellers though no date of publication is given. The title on the ornamental title-page, above a picture of two women attending a young baby, is given as *The Works of Aristotle, the famous Philosopher, in four parts.* It has engravings and from internal evidence, since it mentions for instance the Registrar-General's returns, is probably a mid-nineteenth century edition. The work is divided into four parts: (1) *The Master-Piece,* (2) *the Midwife,* (3) *Aristotle's Book of Problems, with other Astronomers, Astrologers, and Physicians, concerning the state of Man's Body,* and (4) *Displaying the Secrets of Nature, relating to Physiognomy.* At the back a section on venereal disease has been added with the editorial comment that in

> . . . a former edition of this book the venereal disease was omitted. The reasons, however, which at that time induced me to leave it out, have, upon more mature consideration, vanished. Bad consequences, no doubt, may arise from ignorant persons tampering with medicine in this disorder; but the danger from that quarter seeks to be more than balanced by the great and solid advantages which must arise to the patient from an early knowledge of his case . . .[23]

This explanation suggests a serious intention to inform the layman, which is borne out also by the *Advertisement* at the beginning of the volume on the need for a guide for both midwives and mothers-to-be. It states:

> At the present time, when so many of the female sex, in the hour of Nature's extremity, depend solely upon the skill and practical experience in the Midwife, we regard every attempt to assist the female accoucheur in her difficult, and sometimes dangerous operation, as a blessing conferred upon society. . . Another valuable feature of this work is, that it contains important directions for the guidance of child-bearing women during the time of their pregnancy.[24]

The nineteenth-century edition studied seems at best, on the other hand, to be a reprint of out-of-date material on childbirth and other matters drawn from a variety of sources with classical pretensions, yet still using its more serious purpose of providing information as its selling-point.

The use of the term 'master-piece' appears to refer to the process of procreation from marriage to conception and childbirth, symbolised by a woman. As a frontispiece there is an engraving of a nude woman, with a transparent veil from head to foot, standing before a man dressed as a medieval scholar (the author?) writing at a table, and captioned *Aristotle's Master Piece.*[25] The first two sections of this volume, the *Masterpiece* and the *Midwife,* occupy some two hundred pages, and are devoted to a discussion of female anatomy, conception, pregnancy and delivery of the child. There then follow the other sections mentioned above, comprising another one hundred and fifty pages.

Advice is given on marriage and the choice of partner, and it is suggested that marriage is an attractive subject to both sexes 'except to those who subscribe to the principles of Malthus'.[26] Marrying too young, bodily or mental disqualifications, being dazzled by the other's beauty, seeking wealth, lack of candour and uprightness are all listed as false steps towards matrimony. The unequal ages of the partners is regarded as suggesting other motives in one or other 'than the one that should always be predominant at the hymeneal altar'.[27] Emphasis is placed on the virtues and chastity of both the man and the woman, with references to classical figures as examples. Pliny's praise of his wife,[28] and the conduct of both Ulysses and his wife are mentioned,[29] while Alcmena in Plautus' *Amphitruo* is quoted as being a virtuous young woman – a wife 'more precious than rubies'.[30]

There is little in the way of a detailed account of sexual relations, and there is no discussion or advice on the number of pregnancies, their frequency, desirable size of family, or the prevention of conception. It is only on childbirth that the descriptions and anatomical drawings are technical enough to offer information to the layman or woman. The section of *Aristotle's Works* which probably become most notorious for its more explicit information was the *Masterpiece*, sometimes published as a separate tract. The earliest English version in the British Museum Catalogue is that printed for 'W.B.W.' in London in 1694 with the title *Aristotle's Masterpiece, or, The Secrets of Generation displayed in all the parts thereof, etc.* It is listed under 'Aristotle (Doubtful or Supposititious Works) in English', though there is an earlier edition, dated 1690, in the library of the Wellcome Institute for the History of Medicine.[31] D'Arcy Power has suggested that this publication began its career in Western Europe as a folio in Venice in 1503, and first appeared in English in an edition printed by George Bishop in 1583.[32] Widow Orwin produced her edition in London in 1595, and another in Edinburgh the same year. D'Arcy Power listed twenty-five editions from 1684 to 1930, and there may well have been many more. The 1791 edition by The Booksellers, titled *The Works of Aristotle,* begins with the *Complete Masterpiece.*[33] A comparison between these and the mid-nineteenth-century edition suggests a number of interesting lines of argument, indications of changes in approach and attitude by the publishers, editors, and others.

In the mid-nineteenth-century edition this section of *Aristotle's Works* gives an anatomical description of the womb in the pelvic cavity, denoting its neck and main body, the hymen, clitoris, and the ovaries. The right (male) and left (female) concept is set out, whereby different organs of the body are related by their characteristics to their function in reproduction. This was taken from humoral pathology based on Aristotelian and Galenic theories that all matter is composed of the four elements, or qualities, of wet, dry, hot and cold. It is therefore, suggested in the *Masterpiece* that in 'the right side of the cavity, by reason of the heat of the liver, males are conceived; and in the left side, by the coldness of the spleen, females'.[34] The constitution of the male and the female had, of necessity, in this system to be oppositional in order to allow propagation to take place. This is again laid out clearly:

> . . . man is therefore hot and dry, woman cold and moist; he is the agent, she the patient or weaker vessel, that she should be the subject to the office of the man. It is necessary the woman should be of a cold constitution, because in her is required a redundancy of nature for the infant depending upon her.[35]

The menstrual cycle was part of this system or relationship between the elements of hot and cold. Menstrual blood was regarded as the nutrient for the unborn child – otherwise it was 'a monthly flux of excrementitious blood' superfluous to the needs of either.[36] The woman, therefore, must perform this form of expelling or having something of a redundant nature. The failure to menstruate was explained in the *Masterpiece* as being the result of the woman being too hot and therefore all-consuming, and unable to give the matter required for procreation.[37] This nineteenth-century edition thus reiterated at least some remnants of the sixteenth and seventeenth-century – and even earlier – debates on the role of menstruation in procreation, and its relationship to the four elements in the composition of matter.

There follow another fourteen chapters, in the nineteenth-century edition used here, hastily edited and numbered in the wrong sequence, on various conditions and ailments concerning menstruation, the womb, moles and false conceptions, how to tell if a woman has conceived, untimely births, how pregnant women should conduct themselves, labour and delivery of the child and the difficulties which may be encountered. The signs that a woman is carrying a male child are said to be that the child lies on her right side, following the idea mentioned above, and her right breast is harder and plumper with a redder nipple; she is also said to carry a male child higher than a female. For a girl all the signs are on the left side of the mother. The cures given for all ailments are various versions of bleeding, cupping, potions and purges to soothe or expel the 'humours', bathing, pessaries and injections, plasters and poultices, a regulated diet and a stipulated amount of exercise and rest. For inflammation of the womb for instance the cure is given:

> Let the humours flowing to the womb be repelled, for effecting which, after cooling clysters, open a vein in the arm. If she not be enceinte; the day after strike the saphena on both feet, fasten ligatures and cupping-glasses to the arm, and rub the upper part. Purge gently with cassia, rhubarb, and senna two drachms, aniseed one scruple, barleywater a sufficient quantity; make a decoction. At the beginning of disease anoint the privities and reins with oil of roses and quinces; make plasters of plantain, linseed, barley-meal, white of eggs, and, if the pain be vehement, a little opium; ferment the genitals with the decoction of poppy heads.[38]

Most of these 'medicines' were common herbs, although some may have been more unfamiliar or known as being associated with particular trades – for instance fenugreek was used by farriers, and opapanax in soap as a perfume, both often mentioned in this publication. The more serious the patient's condition the larger were the number of ingredients used in the concoctions, a common practice in herbal treatment. The application of herbs internally and externally was a very ancient practice and based on old herbal prescriptions.[39] They covered the most obvious forms of cure or treatment then known, apart from surgery. The herbs and their application may well have scandalised D' Arcy Power, but were they beyond the experience and knowledge of ordinary men and women? Probably not; some of the less well-known ingredients may have been replaced by others in later editions, but the methods of application and their supposed effectiveness probably remained unchanged. The popularity of such a publication may help to explain the survival into the present century of some of the 'remedies' used by women on themselves for various disorders, especially those involving the use of pessaries and immersions, more usually associated with methods used to procure an abortion.

There is, however, no hint in this book about such matters, no mention of how conception may be prevented or avoided, or an abortion procured. The nearest reference to this concerned the various remedies suggested as cures for the late appearance of menstruation, and indeed the emphasis of the whole book is very much to the contrary, giving advice on how to achieve conception and the successful termination of pregnancy with the safe delivery by the midwife of a live child. It was this aspect of *Aristotle's Works* which was much criticised by the early birth controllers in the early decades of the nineteenth century, but presumably it would have remained even more an 'undercover publication' if it had dealt with such things.[40] Popular ideas about abortifacients circulated among women as an oral tradition, probably with even less chance of being written down than had these ideas on pregnancy and childbirth. It is therefore even more difficult for the historian to discover the 'remedies' that formed part of a popular tradition and knowledge. Raspberry-leaf tea, for instance, was often used, especially in rural areas, and is still remembered today by older women as an explanation of a miscarriage – 'she has been at the raspberry-leaf tea'.

The section following the *Masterpiece* in *Aristotle's Works* is the *Midwife: Guide to Child-bearing Women.* This covers very much the same ground as the *Masterpiece* with similar advice and remedies, but gives details of pregnancy month by month with comments on the diet and exercise to which the woman should adhere. Detailed instructions as given for the midwife to observe at the birth of the child, the method of cutting the umbilical cord, the removal of the 'secundine' or afterbirth, and the procedures to follow in cases of difficult labour and delivery. Attention is paid particularly to the delivery of the whole child without severing the head or limbs, a topic which is also covered in Willughby's manuscript on midwifery compiled from his case notes when practising as a doctor in Derby and Stafford from about 1640 to 1670.[41] This may be a comment on the methods of delivery in common use at that time. At the end of this section there is a drawing of a male child in the womb at the ninth month with various parts of the anatomy labelled. Plates showing the process of delivery or birth of the child, as well as the foetus in the womb at each month, are included earlier in the *Masterpiece* section.

The twentieth-century edition studied follows closely these two main sections of this mid-nineteenth-century copy. There is however a marked difference between them and the seventeenth and eighteenth-century editions, in which the *Masterpiece* is much more explicit in not confining the anatomical description to that of the womb and process of pregnancy, but including detailed descriptions of the sex organs of both men and women. In the 1791 edition the *Masterpiece* is followed by a short chapter, 'The Family Physician', dealing with the spitting of blood, worms in children, ointment for the itch and similar topics. The

Experienced Midwife which follows, before continuing with advice on conception, conduct of the woman during pergnancy and the safe delivery of the child, repeats in almost the same detail the descriptions of the sexual organs of men and women and how they function during sexual intercourse. In particular, in the 1690 and 1791 editions, female genitalia are described in detail and compared with the male, the similarities as well as the differences being pointed out, especially in relation to the clitoris:

> The external parts in womens (sic.) privities, or that which is most obvious to the eye at first, commonly called Pudendum, are designed by nature to cover the great orifice; Nature intending that orifice to receive the penis or yard in the act of coition and also to give passage to the urine, and, at the time of the birth, to the child. The use of the wings or knobs, like myrtleberries, are for the security of the internal part, by shutting up the orifice and neck of the bladder, also for delight and pleasure; for, by their swelling up, they cause titillation and delight in those parts, being pressed by the man's yard . . .
>
> The use and action of the clitoris in women, is like that of the penis or yard in men, that is erection; its extreme end being like that of the glands of the man, the seat of greatest pleasure in the act of copulation, so is this of the clitoris in women, and therefore called the sweetness of love, and the fury of venury. [42]

This has all been omitted from the nineteenth and twentieth-century editions consulted, which became much more of a midwife's manual with some additional sections. Steven Marcus, commenting on this feature in the earlier editions, has suggested that their emphasis on female sexuality and its pleasurable aspects was in marked contrast to later more male-orientated publications on such matters, especially those of the nineteenth century.[43] Keith Thomas, making a similar point, suggests that the suppression of details of female sexuality may have occurred earlier, perhaps in the eighteenth century.[44] The 1791 edition already quoted suggests, nevertheless, that editions containing the earlier franker anatomical detail were still in circulation. Certainly D'Arcy Power was in no doubt that the editions he had seen confirmed the view that this section of *Aristotle's Works* should be roundly condemned: 'The *Masterpiece* at its best is a mere catchpenny production written for the prurient-minded and the less said about it the better.'[45] At some stage, and particularly by the mid-nineteenth century, such information on female genitalia and the sources of sexual excitement in the woman were evidently regarded as unnecessary and undesirable for men and women to have. The pleasurable aspects and the direct comparison with male genitalia especially were omitted. The social significance of this may be connected with prevailing concepts of the woman's passive role in procreation, which also had an Aristotelian origin. The anonymous editor of the 1791 edition was quite aware of the possible reaction of some of his readers to this section:

> That the knowledge of the secrets of Nature is too often abused by many persons, I readily grant, and think it very unfortunate that there should be a generation of such profligate persons in the world; but at the same time do aver that this is no objection to this work.[46]

This part of this collection of Aristotelian and other writings appears to be the one which established its prurient reputation. In contrast, it is interesting that none of the editions studied, early or late, give very much information on the sex act itself. There is a section in the 1690 edition offering advice on copulation, but it is carefully stated that 'we shall cloath (sic.) it in that Modest Dress that the Chastest Ears may hear it, without being put to the trouble of a blush'.[47] Wine and music are suggested but not too much to eat or drink: '. . . a little of what is good, and well digested, breeds good Blood, good Blood creates good Spirits, and when a Man is invigorated with a plentiful Stock of such, he is able to do Miracles'.[48] This section ends with a little more advice on these lines. By the nineteenth century even this kind of advice has been deleted, leaving only those sections advising the woman on how to conduct herself, what to eat, what exercise to take, whether to cough, etc. during the nine months of pregnancy.[49]

The late eighteenth-century edition studied is much more forthright yet contains a large element of fun. At the point at which readers might begin to feel embarrassed at the detail being offered, the editor turns to verse and lightens the whole tone of his discourse. For instance, in the detailed sections on male and female genitalia and the similarities, he ends by summing up the situation:

> Thus the woman's secrets I have survey'd
> And let them see how curiously they're made.
> And that, tho' they of different sexes be,
> Yet on the whole they are the same as we.
> For those that have the strictest searchers been,

Find women are but men turn'd outside in:
And then if they but cast their eyes about,
May find they're women with their inside out.[50]

The emphasis here again is on the similarity between the sexes, and the implication is of mutual pleasure.

This edition is also much more explicit on the sex act itself, but this information comes in a section entitled *Aristotle's Last Legacy* printed at the end of this collection. The advice is offered with a light touch giving directions to both sexes on 'how to manage themselves in the Act of Coition or Venereal Embraces'. The editor once more uses verse to explain what should take place. He suggests that the bride and bridegroom prepare themselves by letting 'their animal and vital spirits be powerfully exhilarated by some brisk and generous restoratives. . . survey the beauties of each other, and bear the bright ideas of them in their minds', and then describes the way in which some 'brisk bridegroom' has thought it necessary 'to delineate the scene of their approaching happiness':

I will enjoy thee, now, my fairest; come,
And fly with me to love's Elysium;
Now my unfranchis'd hand on ev'ry side
Shall o'er they naked polish'd iv'ry slide.
Now free as th'ambient air, I will behold
They bearded snow and thy unbraided gold.
No curtain now, tho' of transparent lawn,
Shall be before thy virgin treasure drawn.
Now thy rich mine, to my enquiring eye
Expos'd, shall ready for my mintage lie.
My rudder with they bold hand, like a try'd
And skilful pilot, thou shall steer, and guide
My bark into love's chamber, where it shall
Dance as the bounding waves do rise and fall,
And my tall pinnance in the Cyprian streight
Shall ride at anchor and unlade her freight.[51]

The editor thus overcomes having to explain in descriptive anatomical terms what takes place physically. He goes on to suggest that the man's withdrawal when 'vanquished, (for he must needs be vanquished that has in the encounter lost his artillery)',[52] should be careful, and follows this with advice on sleep for the bride and general repose with no coughing or sneezing to ensure conception.

Whether these more explicit editions were still available at a later date is difficult to tell, although it is quite likely. This particular copy of the 1791 edition is well bound in leather and probably was part of a private library. Other, cheaper, tracts or sections using similar descriptions may have been reprinted for street sales. Certainly, by comparison, the mid-nineteenth-century edition used here is duller, confining itself much more to the matter of conception, pregnancy and childbirth.

What were the origins of this type of publication, and the scientific basis of the knowledge, ideas and remedies it offered?

One of the most interesting aspects of the sixteenth and seventeenth centuries must have been not only the greater understanding of the universe, the knowledge accumulated by and available to scholars,[53] but also its assimilation by and percolation through to other ranks of Western European society. Politicians, theologians and others were conscious of the problems posed by the wider dissemination of knowledge. At the same time ordinary men and women in their daily lives wanted to know about, and have presumably always sought explanations of natural phenomena, the heavenly bodies and their influence on this planet, sources of power and movement, the source of life and the birth of future generations, and the workings of the human body. This need for explanation, and often for what amounted to reassurance, was met by religious doctrines and teachings, by folklore,[54] and perhaps even more by the accumulation of practical experience and observations, handed on from generation to generation, of countless individuals. This was not purely an oral tradition. The wider sale of printed books, tracts, pamphlets, chapbooks, and the like, from the sixteenth century onwards, began to open up opportunities for the growth of a popular literature on a variety of subjects of a scientific and medical nature, including childbirth and midwifery.

Guides to midwives and women generally date probably from the sixteenth century as printed handbooks. Bennett has suggested that there was a considerable increase in the production of medical books in the latter half of the sixteenth century, though not without opposition from those who wished to safeguard the mystery surrounding medical matters by restricting the circulation of medical information, and from those who were probably making a similar point by opposing the printing of such books in the vernacular instead of in Latin.[55] Of particular interest, therefore, were the two types of obstetrical literature being printed at this time – firstly the translations of ancient gynaecological writings compiled as treatises on obstetrics, and secondly popular guides being compiled as treatises for midwives.[56] Needham has suggested that Roesslin's *De Partu Hominis* published in Frankfort in 1532 was probably an example of the first, and that Rueff's *De Conceptu et Generatione Hominis* published in Latin in 1554 was an example of the second. Both of these works were soon translated into English bearing the titles of *The Birth of Mankynde, otherwise called the Woman's Book*, and *The Expert Midwife*,[57] and were re-edited and reprinted many times in following centuries. One of the most influential translations of and commentaries on Aristotle, which was often incorporated into such editions by popularisers, was probably that of Albertus, surnamed Magnus, Bishop of Ratisbon in the thirteenth century.[58] According to Needham this may have been one of the sources of *Aristotle's Works*,[59] and there are references in the later editions to Albertus and his ideas.[60] Lawn, however, has drawn attention to the 'well-nigh inexplicable tangle' of the origins of this type of literature, and the existence of a pseudo-Albertus work which was also a popular gynaecological tract still being printed at a much later date.[61] There are also some similarities to the literature by Trotula on women's diseases, menstruation and pregnancy.

This was possibly one of the most important modern medical sources of information on these topics. It was modern in the sense of being a treatise written by a doctor practising in the eleventh century drawing on the much earlier classical texts of Hippocrates, Soranus, Aristotle and others, and relating their theories with her own experience.[62] The fate of Trotula's work, especially in the sixteenth century, throws light both on the way in which such manuscripts received greater attention at this period and were printed for a wider readership, and also on the re-interpretations, extracting of information from such works, plagiarising and alterations of authorship which occurred as various compilations of this kind of material were edited. The first printed edition of Trotula's manuscript appeared in Strasbourg in 1544 by Schottus, followed by others in Venice in 1547, 1554, 1555 and 1556.[63] Her work forms part of the writings and research of the great school of Salerno. However, in the Wolff edition of 1556, published in Basel, her authorship is suppressed and the credit given to a Roman freedman, Eros or Erotes.[64] Thus her work became part of a mysterious indiscriminate collection of medical data and observations used and mis-used until recently by plagiarists, popularisers and quacks. The role of women medical practitioners and theorists was evidently denied and obscured.

Such reprints in English of older manuscripts and classical texts were in part, until at least the eighteenth century, serious studies or attempts to make known to a wider readership work already available in a particular field such as medicine, anatomy and the natural sciences. Any distinction between professional, scholarly and lay would be quite difficult to make, except perhaps when such material was more obviously used as titillating tracts. Indeed such well-known editors and writers on medical matters as Salmon and Culpeper were associated with versions of *Aristotle's Works.* Fontenelle was another to be regarded as an excellent populariser of science, including theories on the problem of generation.[65] This suggests that while its origins were ancient it received some professional attention as a popular handbook in the seventeenth century, and perhaps then began to pass into a more popular phase of its history, less and less supported by professional opinion and editorship. This raises another question concerning professional versus lay knowledge, although no clear-cut division has been apparent between them until recently. Professional knowledge may then be split between the academic intellectual researcher, writer and philosopher, and the professional practitioner. The latter may well have continued to use well-known treatments and handbooks as were proven in his experience and acceptable to his patients and their concepts of what was happening to them – a familiar problem for the medical profession working today in very different cultures such as in the Third World. This may well have assisted in the survival of Aristotelian and Galenic concepts of matter and generation at the popular level, and of humoral pathology.

It would appear then that a popular literature on natural science and medical matters had clearly begun to develop a printed life of its own. It is possible that it increasingly diverged from the most advanced scientific thought and investigation of the time as the popular manuals tended to adhere to the ancient schools of thought. They were, moreover, based on sixteenth and seventeenth-century re-statements of Aristotelian and Galenic ideas at a time when such ideas were being seriously challenged. Some idea of this can be gained, for instance, from King's discussion of the writings of the Galenist Riverius, who taught at the famous medical school of Montpelier in the early years of the seventeenth century, and of the challenge mounted by Van Helmont, Boyle and others to such teachings.[66] The long-established concept of the four elements, forming the basis of all explanations of natural phenomena, came under attack particularly in intellectual circles, but survived elsewhere. Popular printed manuals on natural science, midwifery and related topics long continued to contain some aspects of Aristotelian concepts of form, matter, sources of life-giving power, etc.

The way in which Aristotelian ideas remained an integral part of these works is strikingly demonstrated in the section of *Aristotle's Works* entitled the *Problems,* which follows the midwifery chapters in the mid-nineteenth century edition. This includes *Aristotle's Book of Problems,* the *Problems of Marcus Antonius Zimara Sanctipertias* and the *Problems of Alexander Aphrodiensias.* D'Arcy Power has stated that the collection purporting to be *Aristotle's Problems* had a wide circulation in Western Europe in the fifteenth and sixteenth centuries,[67] and Lawn has suggested that it was compiled perhaps in the fourteenth or fifteenth century as a popular problem publication, being widely translated throughout Western Europe especially in English, the first edition being printed by Widow Orwin in 1595.[68] The *Problems of Zimara* and the *Problems of Alexander* were often printed with this pseudo-*Aristotle's Problems,* preserving the question and answer form of classical problem literature. The fact that the same or similar questions occur in these two sections suggests that they were to some extent drawn from the same source. They probably formed part of the literature classified as of some Aristotelian origin which was translated in the fifteenth century by Gaza and others.[69] The questions include comments on man's conduct, his wisdom and injustice, and on natural or physical characteristics, particularly the difference between the sexes.

One of the 'problems', for instance, dealt with by Zimara was:

Q. How come women's bodies to be looser, softer and, less than men's; and why do they want hair?

A. By reason of their menses; for with them their superfluities go away, which would produce hair; and thereby the flesh is filled, consequently the veins are more hid in women than in men.[70]

A similar question occurs in *Aristotle's Book of Problems* as printed in this compilation, *Aristotle's Works.*[71] This type of problem and explanation largely fell within the framework of the Aristotelian concept of the constitution of matter by which all matter was defined in terms of varying proportions of the four fundamental qualities of hot, cold, wet and dry, based on the four elements of earth, air, fire and water. The theory had also been combined with the Hippocratic idea of the four humours of blood, phlegm, black bile for melancholy and yellow bile for choler,[72] and questions on these humours occur elsewhere in

Aristotle's Works. Phlegm and bile were common terms used in folk and lay medicine until recent times to describe or explain certain conditions or illnesses.

In this type of popular medical manual the Aristotelian and Galenic ideas of humoral pathology remained the dominant theme. It was an attractive one, since it offered a schematic explanation of biological or natural phenomena easily understandable by the layman or woman. It was simple, with its own integral logic, linking human physical and physiological features with a personality determined by natural phenomena, especially the heavenly bodies; that is, personality was associated with physiognomy and with astrological signs. *Aristotle's Works* included sections on both, that on physiognomy still having some roots at least in Aristotle's own writings.

According to D'Arcy Power,[73] the *Physiognomia* is another spurious work attributed to Aristotle, possibly dating in fact from the third century A.D., and much translated in the sixteenth and seventeenth centuries. The continued publication of this section of *Aristotle's Works* in the late eighteenth and nineteenth centuries is not difficult to understand given the new fashion for physiognomy at that time, and the interest in the work of Lavater relating the human face and human temperament to the influence of the planets and the signs of the zodiac. Lavater's *Essays on Physiognomy* were translated from German into English in the 1780s, and his influence continued for several decades after his death in 1801.[74]

Much that must have puzzled the lay mind was apparently explained away by such systems or compilations of ideas. The explanations and remedies, on the other hand, may not themselves have been of as much importance as the information they contained, for instance on the physical differences and features of the sexes. *Aristotle's Problems* in this popularised version deals with various parts of the body from the head downwards, and poses a number of questions such as for instance, why 'have not men as great paps and breasts as women?', why 'do the paps of young women begin to grow about 13 to 15 years of age?', and why are 'women's paps hard when they are pregnant, and soft at other times?'[75] This information on physical features was probably of greater interest to the uninformed reader than the explanations offered for their existence. There are also questions on infants, including one on why do children 'born in the eighth month for the most part die quickly?' Information given through the medium of questions regarding the higher mortality of babies born at the eighth month of pregnancy was again probably more helpful than the explanation given that such children were called 'the children of the moon', because 'the moon is a cold planet, which has dominion over the child, and therefore doth bind it with its coldness, which is the cause of its death'.[76] It would appear that the relevance of the scientific information to popular belief may have become less and less important, and that it was the hard, practical, observable information which was noted. It may be that such publications were mainly read for this purpose, the explanations offered adding to the mystery rather than actually explaining why and how things occurred.

In particular the information and explanations were given as comments on phenomena, albeit natural phenomena. This may have served a purpose in reducing fears of the unknown or apparently inexplicable. The section on monsters is an example, and this chapter of *Aristotle's Works* may appear to be little more than pandering to an interest in the macabre. On the other hand some comment on monsters, often here termed more kindly as the 'vagaries of nature',[77] was usual in manuals on obstetrics from the sixteenth century onwards. This short section on monsters is in no way horrific and is simply a description with illustrations of unusual examples which had been documented elsewhere. Each is given a date and place of origin, mainly somewhere in Western Europe, and was probably drawn from Ambroise Pare's *Chyrugerie* printed in 1579.[78] There is no suggestion that monsters were the work of the devil or a consequence of the sins of the parents, but that they simply reflect the Aristotelian concept of form in generation operating on matter to shape it, and in the case of monsters not completely mastering the matter. There is also some comment on monsters in the sections of *Aristotle's Works* known as the *Problems.* What would a Victorian reader make of this?

Experience of deformities in newborn children must have been more widespread than in our own time where the process of birth and delivery of the child is institutionalised and observed almost entirely by medically trained personnel. When the birth took place within the family home with the mother assisted by famale relatives and neighbours, physical abnormalities, sometimes of an extensive kind, could be witnessed. The monsters dealt with in popular manuals such as *Aristotle's Works* were romanticised and exaggerated examples. Such information may have added to the fears of a woman for her unborn child, while at the same time it gave her some forewarning of its possible lack of physical perfection, and this may have been the intention of this section.

It is only really possible to suggest, rather than to assert, the impact on and the use made by the readership of such information. Other studies of this publication have made little comment on its social significance, and have perhaps too easily assumed that its readership was the 'prurient-minded'. They have instead attempted to trace the classical and pseudo-classical origins. Where comments have been made by the medical profession, they, as to be expected, have stressed its lack of relevance and possible dangers as a modern medical reference book. Beall, as an historian, has suggested that this work is an example of the popular medical literature available in North America in the eighteenth and early nineteenth centuries, drawing 'indiscriminately from writers of ancient Greece and Rome; from the works of sixteenth, seventeenth, and eighteenth-century medical writers; and from the vast accretions of European folklore'.79 In his view the Aristotelian content is possibly negligible and he therefore concentrates on the probable English editors, and on the various editions which appeared in North America between 1760 and 1840 to indicate its popularity. There is little discussion of the contents of these different editions, and little attempt to explain the significance of this work being associated in North America at this period with Aristotelian teachings on generation and related topics.

The wide circulation of this publication attracted the attention of D'Arcy Power in his studies of medical history, and he was especially concerned at its continued publication in the twentieth century.80 He particularly noted the perpetuation of myths, ancient theories and pseudo-medical advice and treatment, and found their reprinting explicable only by their interest for the prurient-minded. He has shown his distaste to the more modern reprints as being:

> . . . a hoary old debauchee acknowledged by no one. In fact, it is so disreputable that I had some difficulty in bringing myself to buy a copy. It is sold only in those shops which are devoted to contraceptives and I thought that if my numerous friends saw me going in or met me coming out my object would certainly be misinterpreted . . . I cannot think who now buys or reads it, and yet it seems to have a large and constant sale. I have now knowledge of sixty-six editions and there were at least ten copies in the shop where I bought this one, and if there are two hundred such shops in London alone there must be two thousand copies in circulation. It is continually being reprinted so that the demand seems to remain constant. There must be a large class of person in England possessed of prurient minds and so uneducated that the pseudo-science of the

middle ages still appeals to them.[81]

He too has little to say about the changes in content, which were made from time to time, their significance in the debate on Aristotelian ideas on generation which continued into the nineteenth century, and the links with popular ideas about such matters. An attempt will now be made to discuss the way in which ideas were transmitted and popularised.

One of the most fascinating features of *Aristotle's Works* is the inclusion of some comment on the debate on generation which had continued for centuries. As Preus has suggested in his analysis of the *Generation of Animals,* Aristotle was trying to solve 'a group of problems which are central both for biology and for Aristotle's philosophical system', that is, a concern with how new life begins and with the metaphysical importance of that explanation of animal generation.[82] The theoretical solution Aristotle offered depended essentially on drawing a distinction between potentiality and actuality in the change from non-being to being, and this had important physical, and therefore, scientific implications. What has survived in the popularised version of *Aristotle's Works* is a truncated and simplified explanation of animal generation, assigning particular roles to the two sexes. While this may be a travesty of Aristotle's metaphysical analysis, it has had important social implications.

It was in the seventeenth century, in particular, that Aristotle's theories on generation began to be re-assessed, not least as a result of the work of William Harvey in the middle decades of the century.[83] It is possible that, at that time, writings on midwifery and childbirth for more popular consumption reflected, to some extent, this debate on generation. An analysis of the seventeenth-century edition, printed by 'F.L.' for 'J.How' in London in 1690, suggests this. It bears the title *Aristotle's Masterpiece: or, The Secrets of Generation Displayed in all the Parts thereof,* and its contents are said to be 'very necessary for all Midwives, Nurses, and Young Married Women'. It begins with an explanation of the creation of the world, and of procreation and marriage as necessary for the continuation of mankind, and follows with a discussion on the begetting of a male or female child, linking this with the woman sleeping on her left or right side after intercourse.[84] The role of the man and the woman in generation is then explained, based on the presence of the two principles, the active and the passive:

The Active is the Man's Seed, which is elaborated in the Testicles

> out of the Arterial Blood and Animal Spirits. The Passive Principle, is an *Ovum* or Egg, impregnated by the Man's Seed. For to say that Woman has true Seed, is false and erroneous. But the manner of Conception is thus. The most Spirituous part of Man's Seed, in the act of Generation, reaching up to the Ovanium or Testicles of the Woman (which contain divers Eggs, sometimes more, sometimes fewer) fecundates one of them, which being conveyed by the Oviducts to the bottom of the Womb, presently begins to swell and grow bigger. . .[85]

This is a curiously modern approach, modern that is in its terminology and very similar to a footnote Hugh Chamberlen added to his version of generation in his translation of Mauriceau's work on midwifery published in 1683.[86] Needham has suggested this was 'enlightened common sense'[87] on the part of Chamberlen, and the use in the *Masterpeice* of the term 'impregnated' should perhaps be viewed in the same way. Scientists stimulated by Harvey's work on generation had continued their observations on the conveyance of the fertilised egg to the womb, but fertilisation remained imperfectly understood for more than another century, and therefore too much importance should not be attached to this terminology. This passage, on the other hand, does appear to amalgamate the more advanced concepts of generation of the time with the older concepts of the active and passive principles: that is the male being active and the female passive. The concept of the two principles had allowed for the separation of the male's active role in generation and his physical role in copulation; that is, it was thought, the matter present in the womb could be activated by the male without physical contact with the male's seed necessarily taking place. His was thought to be the life-giving force in the more spirituous sense, giving form to the passive matter contributed by the female and thereby allowing for the possibility of a virgin birth.[88] Some element of this idea remains in the seventeenth-century version of generation by the reference to the 'most Spirituous part of Man's Seed'. As the passage quoted above makes clear, the two seed or Epicurean concept was refuted, however, in favour of the idea that the woman's seed was analogous to eggs found in other species which had to be impregnated by the male seed. Physical contact, impregnation, was now regarded as essential for fertilisation to occur, leading to theories of both male and female contributions to the life-giving process in some physical form.

The nature of the contribution of each sex remained a matter of controversy, leading to the debate about preformation in the eighteenth century between the two schools of the ovists and the animalculists. The former emphasised the predominance of the female physical contribution, the latter the male.[89] In the seventeenth-century version the concept of the active and passive principles was additionally retained in some form. The function of the female egg was still being confused with the ancient idea of the female contributing the inert matter, its potential only realised by being activated by the male seed; that is, it was the fertilised egg which descended rather than the modern view of the egg independently descending and being fertilised only after ovulation. The ancient view thereby maintained the emphasis on the male role of activating the egg or female seed which could only then move or descent to the womb.

This short explanation of generation in the 1690 edition may be regarded as an interesting transmission statement, revealing the confusion of new and of old ideas existing at the end of the seventeenth century. It also indicates some editing, or up-dating, of the publication – of which there is more evidence in the Victorian version, where the passage quoted above is repeated in substantially the same terms, and is classified as being the 'modern' view. The contrast is then made with the older or ancient theory; that is, the two seed theory whereby 'the seed of man is the principal efficient and beginning of action, motion, and generation',[90] but that the woman also produces seed. This raises the problem of assigning a role to each of the seeds, resolved somewhat unsatisfactorily in this edition by assuming that 'since nature forms nothing in vain, it must be granted they (the woman's "seminal vessels") were made for use of seed and procreation, and fixed in their proper places, to operate, and contribute virtue and efficiency to the seed'.[91] The editor of the nineteenth-century version states that he will not himself become a party to this controversy, and simply goes on to note that the modern view stems from the fact that the woman's seed is 'like those (the eggs) of fowls and other creatures', which are fertilised by the man's seed. The editor points out how the modern version subscribes to the view that the male seed is the active principle in generation, and that the ovum or the egg is the passive principle. There still remains, therefore, in the 'modern' view, as given in the Victorian edition, this fusion of the ancient or Aristotelian view of two principles in generation – the man's active and the woman's passive role – with the new or modern idea of the male seed impregnating the female seed or egg. That the editor of this version remained undecided in his views is scarcely surprising since von Baer's work on the mamalian ovum was only just becoming known and the medical profession was still undecided about the contribution of the two sexes in generation. A few decades later a comment on the state of this controversy noted that the 'old conception of the male influence lingered persistently'.[92] There is still some evidence in the late seventeenth century-edition that the woman as well as the man was thought to have some vital fluid. The later version has sometimes been used symbolically as evidence of man's superiority in giving this vital, life-giving fluid to the woman who does not possess it – again a reversion to the Aristotelian concept.

Histories of theories of generation reveal the long evolution of our knowledge and understanding of what takes place at conception.[93] The various reprints and editions of *Aristotle's Works* add another dimension to this process – the way in which scientific ideas and information become part of popular literature and knowledge. This publication is an example of how, in the modern era of printing, popular versions of scientific ideas were produced and circulated, slowly developing a life of their own which possibly lasted long after the ideas had been scientifically questioned. Moreover, periodic re-editing introduced some indications of current scientific debate. Popular beliefs about health and disease, life and death and the like were clearly not static. The way they evolve and their sources of new ideas must, in part, have been dependent on advances made in professional science and medicine.

This appears to be a process whereby initially there exists at a particular time, a body of well-established ideas about the origins of life, causes of good health and disease, etc., forming at the popular level a system of knowledge. The ideas are rooted in a particular system of scientific principles and re-interpreted, at the practical level, by everyday usage and custom. There impinges on the old system of principles new scientific ideas – such as those on generation. New knowledge is not only taken up and debated at the professional level, but is also interpreted at the popular level. Thus new knowledge is somehow transmitted and made intelligible to, for and by the layman himself. This new knowledge in turn must relate to current concepts and established popular ideas, either by making it intelligible and socially acceptable within the framework of the old system of knowledge, or by involving a major shift in ideas to the new principles – a shift which is itself made acceptable and preferable.

Past ideas which may be condemned by scientists and the medical profession as out of date may remain important for much longer as part of popular understanding of science, and continue to be related with the new. There may be no clear-cut transfer to the new at the popular level, but probably an extended transition which lacks the sharpness of the conflict which occurs at the expert level between adherents of different schools of thought. What is being tentatively suggested is that there is some kind of social process of interpretation and acceptance to popularise new ideas and to absorb new principles, which integrate or interact with the established body of popular knowledge. This evolutionary process continues from one generation to the next. How this happens and what interaction occurs is difficult to trace: crudely expressed, a fusion of traditional myths with new discoveries, a process of assimilation, can be imagined.

This assimilation of old and new ideas has been complicated by the popular version having a social purpose, being designed to inform men and women within a particular intellectual and social climate, and having to conform to that climate. Such popular works attempted, therefore, to answer or comment on questions of interest and significance at the time. In the sixteenth and seventeenth centuries these were explanations of physical characteristics, human reproduction and inheritance of features, virgin birth, conception of a male child, etc., and the relationship of such matters to the external phenomena beyond human control, such as the planets and stars. They thus reflected the values of the society they were produced to inform, and the ideas were to some degree rendered acceptable to that society. Indeed the system evolved so as to relate the three most obvious or visual aspects of life and the universe – the state of the body, the individual's temperament and the heavens. This question of acceptability must have been especially important when the subject matter concerned sexual relations and the birth of the next generation, and therefore also involved the control of social behaviour, particularly that of women.

How successfully this was done and how far *Aristotle's Works* was an 'acceptable' publication openly read in the centuries before the Victorian age is difficult to determine. There is also the question of the continued social acceptability of such a publication at a later stage of its history when the contents are more clearly outdated. At a more undercover level the *Works* appear to have remained very well known. A partial explanation is to be found in the different versions where the editor has added or excluded material – as for example on venereal disease. The cautious comments of the editor of the mid-nineteenth-century edition on the female egg theory is a further example of where his views may intrude on attempts to understand popular ideas. The process of editing by individuals may reflect to some degree changes in social outlook, or differing attitudes towards new ideas. Such publications are not necessarily, therefore, an accurate guide to people's feelings, responses and attitudes towards certain phenomena. Nonetheless they provide an insight into the system of ideas which was repeatedly presented to ordinary people. Did the ideas thus presented remain unquestioned? Much more likely perhaps was an instinctive degree of acceptance, almost without any positive act of decision-making. How useful, for example, would a woman find such a publication?

Although such a publication assumes an ability to read, assisted in some editions by illustrations, there may also have been some general reassurance and interest among those who could not, from knowing that a book existed on subjects of particular importance and intimate concern to women. Extracts quoted from it may have confirmed views already held or practices attempted, or at least have borne some resemblance to them. Very evident in the text is the mystery element – mystery in the sense of wonder in the exactness, even inevitability, of the processes discussed, and their links with a wider cosmos, the planets, signs of the zodiac, and the thoughts of great philosophers of the past. There is, furthermore, a practical, down-to-earth approach in this compilation – no moralising except for the short section in some editions on the choice of a marriage partner. Otherwise the advice is physical and advisory at a practical level. There is clear evidence of an awareness of the social role of female sexuality; the denial of its existence in later editions formed an important control over sexual behaviour.

Yet again, there is a particular feature of this type of popular literature which is more difficult to elucidate. It is almost too exact in the imprecision or ineffectiveness of much of its advice, and this stems from lack of thought and explanation rather than cogency or simplicity. In its entirety it can be seen as a particular explanation of the order of things, of all matter and of their interrelationships. For the reader the factual evidence rather than the explanation was of crucial importance. This type of literature did not promote thought, or reflection, but simply offered, among other material, a guide to physical matters concerning conception, pregnancy and childbirth. Probably Bourne's analysis of the changes which had taken place in the village by the early years of this century has come nearest in attempting to explain this low level of mental exertion demanded of the reader – a phenomenon which had not just applied to printed material but to a whole way of looking at life.94 Therefore, *Aristotle's Works* is valuable as an example of the type of widely available literature from which were formed the ideas, perceptions and attitudes that gave them cultural determination, roots and origins. It is almost impossible to determine how they were used and interpreted practically in everyday life. The way in which one notion was linked with another, the system of connected notions offered to the reader, these must have had a powerful impact on ordinary people's perception of the world. This system may, in time, have acted 'in lieu' of an explanation, being set out as a 'given', as almost a 'law' of nature from which certain consequences flowed. Apart from offering some kind of placebo, or substitute for thought, such literature must have had the more fundamental effect of denying the need for any form of reflection, or for additional individual thought. The cultural significance of this must have been very important, especially in the field of medicine where the layman was often seen as being subordinate to the professional, and particularly when the topics concerned the origins of life, conception and the delivery of the live child, and much of the information remained part of popular knowledge for centuries. This information was only imperfectly and very inadequately challenged by alternative professionally produced popular sources, and this only in recent times.

Thus it is suggested that such a publication as *Aristotle's Works*, by remaining for centuries a popular manual, provides a barometer of ideas on sexual relations and childbirth. It gives the historian an insight into the way in which popular scientific and medical knowledge has evolved over the centuries, amalgamating old ideas with the new, and rendering them both socially acceptable, in so far as such topics were acceptable at all for public discussion for generations of ordinary men and women. This analysis can only be regarded as a tentative beginning to the study of the complex process of the transmission of ideas and scientific principles from one generation to another, their popularisation, and the attitudes derived from them. In earlier centuries it may well be that *Aristotle's Works* was a popular handbook in the broadest sense, read by all who could read and by anyone interested for any reason in such material, but in the late nineteenth century, in particular, it probably began to attract a much more general working-class readership. The concern is thus with collective behaviour, and with widespread attitudes towards and general understanding of knowledge provided by the professional and the privileged elite, and how the working-class came to absorb or reject such information in their own lives.

Notes

1. K. Thomas, *Religion and the Decline of Magic. Studies in Popular Beliefs in Sixteenth and Seventeenth Century England*, London, 1971
2. A. Macfarlane, *Witchcraft in Tudor and Stuart England*, London, 1970.

3. See for instance, H.F. Kearney, 'Puritanism, Capitalism and the Scientific Revolution', *Past and Present,* no. 28, 1964, 81-101.
4. C.Hill, 'Puritanism, Capitalism and the Scientific Revolution', *Past and Present,* no. 29, 1964, 88-97.
5. T.K. Rabb, 'Puritanism and Science: Problems of Definitions', *Past and Present,* no. 31, 1965, 126 footnote.
6. See in particular, T.S. Kuhn, *The Structure of Scientific Revolutions,* 2nd edn., Chicago, 1970.
7. *Ibid.,* pp. 2-3.
8. There is an interesting eighteenth-century example of such a condemnation of Plato and Aristotle in W. Black's *An Historical Sketch of Medicine and Surgery from their origin to the present* (London, 1782, pp. 38-9), made indirectly by Black using what he terms Lord Bolingborke's 'sentiments'.
9. Thomas, *op. cit.,* p. 5.
10. For a particularly informative study of this problem literature see B. Lawn, *The Salernitan Question; an Introduction to the History of Medieval and Renaissance Problem Literature,* Oxford, 1963.
11. For example, the announcement in a local Scottish newspaper of the birth of a child may still result in the parents receiving an unsolicited copy of this book. There is some evidence that the work is today being passed from mothers to daughters as their way of explaining sexual matters.
12. M. Sadler, *Forlorn Sunset,* London, 1947, p. 412.
13. J. Needham, *A History of Embryology,* New York, 1929, p. 92.
14. A.L. Rowse, *A Cornishman at Oxford,* London, 1965, p. 196.
15. A.L. Peck, *Aristotle's Generation of Animals,* London, 1953, p. v, footnote.
16. Sarah Hickney (afterwards Mrs Ellis), *The Women of England,* 1st edn., London 1839; *Daughters of England,* 1st ed., London 1845. She married in 1837 William Ellis, who became chief foreign secretary of the London Missionary Society. See the entry for both under William Ellis in the *Dictionary of National Biography, vi,* 714-15.
17. C.L. Powell, *English Domestic Relations, 1487-1653,* New York, 1917. See also A. Adburgham, *Women in Print; Writing Women and Women's Magazines from the Restoration to the Accession of Queen Victoria,* London, 1972.
18. I am grateful to Ann Roberts for her assistance on this point. See her *Feeding and Mortality in the Early Months of Life: Changes in Medical Opinion and Popular Practice, 1850-1900,* PhD thesis, University of Hull, 1975.
19. S. Hale, *New Household Receipt-Book,* London, 1854, p. 345.
20. W. Buchan, *Domestic Medicine; or, the Family Physician. . .chiefly calculated to recommend proper attention to regimen and simple medicines,* Edinburgh, 1769. Many editions were published in this country and on the continent. Sergey Aksakov refers to his mother consulting her copy of Buchan in an account of his childhood in Russia. A. Brown (trans.), *Years of Childhood,* 1858, New York, 1960, pp. 9-10, 15-16 and 30-3. I am grateful to Dr. J.W. Thompson of the University of Hull for this reference.
21. This phrase appears on the title page of the 1802 Edinburgh edition.
22. *Ibid.,* p. 569.
23. *Aristotle's Works* (*c.* 1850 edn.), p. 9.
24. *Ibid.* This *Advertisement* appears between the title-page and the list of contents.
25. A similar frontispiece appears in a twentieth-century edition, *c,* 1920, but a veil has been drawn aside.
26. *Aristotle's Works* (*c.* 1850 ed.), p. 9.

27. *Ibid.*, p.10.
28. *Ibid.*, p. 24.
29. *Ibid.*, p. 28.
30. *Ibid.*, p. 29.
31. *Aristotle's Masterpiece; or, the Secrets of Generation Displayed in all the Parts thereof*, printed by 'F.L.' for 'J. How', London 1690. The Index Society, *Short-title Catalogue of Books printed in England, Scotland, Ireland, Wales and British America and of other English Books printed in other countries, 1641-1700,* New York, 1945, gives an earlier version, published in 1684 for J. How.
32. D'Arcy Power, *The Foundations of Medical History*, Baltimore, 1931, p. 168.
33. I am grateful to A.R. Michell of the University of Hull for kindly loaning me a copy of this edition.
34. *Aristotle's Works* (*c.* 1850 edn.), p. 42.
35. *Ibid.*, p. 43.
36. *Ibid.*, pp. 42-3.
37. *Ibid.*, p. 45.
38. *Ibid.*, p. 65.
39. There were, for instance, one or two such herbals translated into old English from the Greek and Latin in the tenth century. These include a similar range of treatment or cures. See A.C. Crombie, 'Science', in A.L. Poole (ed.), *Medieval England,* Oxford, 1958, vol. II, pp. 575-7.
40. I am grateful to Angus McLaren for this information.
41. P. Willughby, *Observations in Midwifery* (edited from the original MSS, by Henry Blenkinsop, 1863, with a new introduction by J.L. Thornton), Wakefield, 1972, pp. 150 and 161-3. For a history of midwifery, see H. Graham, *Eternal Eve,* London, 1950; J.H. Aveling, *English Midwives; their history and prospects* (reprint of 1872 edn.), London, 1967. For a history of the profession see J.E. Donnison, *The Development of the Profession of Midwife in England, 1750-1902,* PhD thesis, University of London, 1974.
42. *The Works of Aristotle* (1791 edn), p. 15, and a further more detailed description on similar lines on pp. 110-12 in the *Experienced Midwife* section. These follow closely the same passages as in the 1690 edition.
43. S. Marcus, *The Other Victorians,* Corgi ed., London 1969, p.29 footnote.
44. Thomas, *op. cit.*, p. 569.
45. Power, *op. cit.*, p. 168
46. *Aristotle's Works* (1791 edn.), p. 2.
47. *Aristotle's Masterpiece* (1690 edn.), p. 173.
48. *Ibid.*, pp. 173-4
49. *Aristotle's Works* (*c.* 1850 edn.), p. 78.
50. *The Works of Aristotle* (1791 edn.), p. 15.
51. *Ibid.*, p. 389. This may be the origins of all those sea scenes of rolling waves used euphemistically in old films as the lovers embrased!
52. *Ibid.*
53. See for instance, W.P.D. Wightman, *Science in a Renaissance Society,* Kibdibm 1972.
54. There is an interesting study of what the author calls 'the mutual interplay of two great human attitudes, scientific and religious, at a specific place and time' in P.H. Kocher, *Science and Religion in Elizabethan England,* New York, 1969.
55. H.S. Bennett, *English Books and Readers, 1558-1603,* Cambridge, 1965, pp. 179-81.
56. Needham, *op. cit.*, pp. 109-12.

57. *Ibid.*, p. 112. See also W.S.C. Copeman, *Doctors and Disease in Tudor Times*, London, 1960, p. 48; and Graham, *op. cit.*, pp. 81 and 139-47. There is some discrepancy as to the date of the original German edition and the first English translation: Graham gives 1532 and 1540 respectively, whereas Copeman suggests 1513 and 1540, and Needham gives the date 1545 as the date of the English edition produced by Thomas Raynold (or Raynalde) as his own work.
58. Needham, *op. cit.*, pp. 89-91.
59. *Ibid.*, p. 92.
60. See, for instance, *Aristotle's Works* (*c.* 1850 edn.), pp. 244-5. For a short but useful comment on Albertus see J. Carter and P.H. Muir (eds.), *A Descriptive Catalogue Illustrating the Impact of Print on the Evolution of Western Civilisation during Five Centuries*, Cambridge, 1967, pp. 10-11.
61. Lawn, *op. cit.*
62. Trotula of Salerno, *The Diseases of Women* (trans. by E. Mason-Hohl, 1940). I am grateful to Susan Groag Bell of the University of Santa Clara, California, for this information and reference.
63. *Ibid.*, p. vii.
64. *Ibid.*, p. x (Foreward by Kate Campbell Hurd-Mead).
65. A.F. Corcos, 'Fontenelle and the problem of generation in the eighteenth century', *Journal of the History of Biology, 4*, 1971, 363-72.
66. L.S. King, *The Road to Medical Enlightenment, 1650-1695*, London and New York, 1970, especially chap. two.
67. Power, *op. cit.*, pp. 149-62.
68. Lawn, *op. cit.*, pp. 99-100.
69. S.D. Wingate, *The Mediaeval Latin Versions of the Aristotelian Scientific Corpus, with Special Reference to the Biological Works*, London, 1931, p. 127. See also A.L. Peek's account of translations of Aristotle's zoological works in his 'Introduction' to his translations of Aristotle's *Parts of Animals*, London, 1937, pp. 39-44.
70. *Aristotle's Works* (*c.* 1850 edn.), p. 259.
71. *Ibid.*, p. 206.
72. For further discussions of these ideas see C. Singer, *The Evolution of Anatomy*, London, 1925, pp. 27-8; C.H. Haskins, *Studies in the History of Mediaeval Science*, New York and London, 1960, pp. 92-6. There is also a useful account of the humoral theory and its origins in D.M. Needham, *Machina Carnis: the biochemistry of muscular contraction in its historical development*, Cambridge, 1971, cap. one.
73. Power, *op. cit.*, p. 164.
74. J. Graham, 'Lavater's physiognomy in England', *Journal of the History of Ideas, 22*, 1961, 561-72.
75. *Aristotle's Works* (*c.* 1850 edn.), pp. 229-32.
76. *Ibid.*, p. 245.
77. *Ibid.*, p. 34.
78. C.J.S. Thompson, *The Mystery and Lore of Monsters*, London, 1930, especially chap. five.
79. Otho T. Beall, '*Aristotle's Masterpiece* in America: a Landmark in the Folklore of Medicine', *William and Mary Quarterly, 20*, 1963, 207-22.
80. Power, *op. cit.*
81. *Ibid.*, p. 147.
82. A. Preus, 'Science and philosophy in Aristotle's *Generation of Animals*', *Journal of the History of Biology, 3*, 1970, 1.
83. For assessments of Harvey's work on generation see J. Needham, *op. cit.*, pp. 133-53; A.W. Meyer, *An Analysis of the* De Generatione Animalium

of William Harvey, London, 1936; G. Keynes, *The Life of William Harvey*, Oxford, 1966; and E. Gasking, *Investigations into Generation, 1651-1828*, London, 1967, especially chap. two. Much of this work is reviewed in F. B. Churchill, 'The history of embryology as intellectual history', *Journal of the History of Biology*, *3*, 1970, 155-81.

84. *Supra*, p. 65.
85. *Aristotle's Masterpiece: or, The Secrets of Generation Displayed in all the Parts therof*, London, 1690, p. 15.
86. J. Needham, *op. cit.*, p. 210.
87. *Ibid.*, p. 209.
88. See H.A. Oberman, *The Harvest of Medieval Theology. Gabriel Biel and late Medieval Nominalism*, Cambridge (Mass.), 1963, chap. nine for some discussion on Mariology and the Immaculate Conception in the medieval tradition, including some comments on the role of the mother in the creation of the child, pp. 288-9.
89. C. Singer, *A History of Biology*, London, 1959, pp. 497-500; P.J. Bowler, 'Preformation and pre-existence in the seventeenth century', *Journal of the History of Biology*, *4*, 1971, 221-44; and J. Needham, *op. cit.* especially chap. four.
90. *Aristotle's Works* (*c.*1850 edn.), p. 91.
91. *Ibid.*
92. P. Geddes and J.A. Thompson, *The Evolution of Sex*, London, 1901, p. 170.
93. H. Graham, *op. cit.*, Gasking, *op. cit.*, and also F.J. Cole, *Early Theories of Sexual Generation*, Oxford, 1930.
94. George Bourne, *Change in the Villiage*, London, 1912, especially chap. fourteen.

3 THE EARLY BIRTH CONTROL MOVEMENT: AN EXAMPLE OF MEDICAL SELF-HELP

Angus McLaren

The story of the emergence of the birth control movement in Britain and the United States in the 1820s and 1830s has been told many times.[1] Attention has been traditionally focused on the economic theories of the early neo-Malthusians; what has however not been fully appreciated is that their activity was part of a widespread nineteenth-century interest in the search for a common man's medicine. A host of self-help medical movements sprang up in the first half of the century combating alcoholism, gluttony, folly in dress and a variety of other ills. These movements shared both the belief that the layman could take preventive measures to ward off most physical complaints and the suspicion that the medical profession either could not or would not instruct him in such measures.[2]

This essay attempts to cast a fresh light on the birth control movement of the 1820s and 1830s by treating it as yet another self-help medical movement. The economic and moral arguments of the movement's advocates have been set aside: rather has attention been focused on the belief that illness was caused by ignorance – in particular that the illnesses associated with repeated unwanted pregnancies and unnecessarily large families were a consequence of an ignorance of contraception. The essay may be divided into three sections: the first deals with those men who had a professional interest in maintaining and exploiting the medical ignorance of the public – the purveyors of handbooks of sexual folklore and quack medications. The second section sketches out the response of the medical profession to the issue of birth control in the first half of the nineteenth century, and the final section presents the birth controllers' arguments in favour of contraception and shows how they formed part of a more general belief in medical self-help.

The birth controllers were, of course, not the first men to provide the public with information on the question of sexuality. In the first half of the nineteenth century there already existed a large popular literature dealing with reproduction. In the first place there was the folklore of sexual knowledge that was finding its way into print. The texts that enjoyed the widest circulation were the series of little books known as *Aristotle's Works.* A London doctor lamented the fact that in the 1830s it was '. . . in great circulation, though replete with error and obscenity from beginning to end'.[3] It has been estimated that close to a hundred editions were published in both the United States and Britain in the latter half of the eighteenth and the first half of the nineteenth centuries.[4] These tracts consisted of a pot-pourri of sexual myths and popular medical beliefs drawn together by seventeenth-century hacks. At least a few of the eighteenth-century editions recognised '. . . that there are some that desire not to have children, and yet are very fond of nocturnal Embraces. . .' but the avowed purpose of these tracts was to explain how to achieve a prolific coition.[5] The reader in search of an accurate portrayal of the process of reproduction would find little useful information but a compendium of the traditional taboos and myths associated with childbearing. Individual chapters dealt with such questions as the use of aphrodisiacs, the predetermination of the sex of offspring, the birth of monsters, and the cures for barrenness. The *Works of Aristotle* and similar publications were medically useless, but their popularity demonstrated, if such demonstration were needed, the popular demand for information on the process of procreation.[6]

This demand was met, in the second place, by a huge outpouring in the late eighteenth and early nineteenth centuries of pamphlets and tracts produced by quacks and charlatans to advertise their wares. A contributor to the *Medical Times* complained in 1839:

> Handbills of the most disgusting character are thrust into the hands of all who venture into public thoroughfares – and thus the eye of female delicacy and innocence is insulted, and the mind of youth defiled, by a detail of the filthy pretensions of these public nuisances.[7]

Such was the concern of the medical profession at the circulation of 'scandalous' quack information in the popular press that it sought to curb such publications through the establishment of the 'Union for the Discouragement of Vicious Advertisements'.[8]

Much of the quack literature has been lost but the more substantial of their tracts and pamphlets give a clear idea of their message. There was, for example, John Leake's *Dissertation on the Properties and Efficiency of the Lisbon Diet-Drink and its Extract in the Cure of Venereal Disease* (1780), James Graham's *A Lecture on the Generation, Increase and Improvement of the Human Species* (1780), Isaac Swainson's *An Account of Cures by Velnos' Vegetable Syrup* (1792),

J. Hodson's, *Nature's Assistant* (1795), William Brodum's *A Guide to Old Age or, A Cure for the Indiscretions of Youth* (1795) and his *To the Nervous, Consumptive and those of Debilitated Constitutions* (1797), Samuel Soloman's *A Guide to Health* (1800), E. Senate's *The Medical Monitor, Containing Observations on the Effects of Early Dissipation* (1810), John Lignum's *A Treatise on Venereal and Syphilitic Diseases* (1819), Gross and Company's *The Aegis of Life* (1830) and their *Hygaeiana, A non-Medical Analysis of the Complaints Incidental to Females* (1830), J.L. Curtis and Company, *Manhood* (1840), J. Jordan and Company, *Human Frailty: Embracing Remarks . . . on the Disease Caused by the Abuses of the Reproductive Functions* (1842), R. and L. Perry and Company, *The Secret Friend* (1845), R. and J. Brody and Company, *The Secret Companion* (1845), Dr Ricord's *Essence of Life* (1860), and Dr Paris' *Treatise on Nervous Debility* (1861). Almost all these works followed the same plan. They provided firstly, a terrifying account of the innumerable diseases which were a consequence of 'evil habits' and 'sexual excesses', secondly a description of the miraculous effects obtained in combating such complaints by the consumption of the quack's potion, and finally a number of letters from satisfied customers testifying to the amazing qualities of the product in question. The publications of Gross and Company were typical of this literature, promising to cure debility caused by 'excessive indulgence in venereal engagements', abstinence, nocturnal emissions, venereal disease, constitutional imbecility, peculiar formation, intensive study, long residence in tropical climates, and masturbation.

The increasing number of speudo-scientific handbills and pamphlets produced by quacks was an indication of the expansion of publishing facilities and the appearance of new advertising schemes. In the eighteenth century quacks limited their propaganda to the well-off; in the nineteenth they shifted their attention to the new urban work force. Dr Andrew Ure was to declare that:

> Nothing strikes the eye of a stranger more in Manchester than the swarms of empirical practitioners of medicine. Nearly a dozen of them may be found clustered together in one of the main streets; all prepared with drastic pills and alternative potions to prey upon credulous spinners.[9]

The circulation of the quacks' literature was in addition an indication of the public's desire for at least some type of instruction on procreation. Only the briefest mention of generation was contained in the respectable popular medical texts such as John Wesley's *Primitive Physick* (1747) or William Buchan's *Domestic Medicine* (1769). This would be as true for serious nineteenth-century works such as Andrew Combe's *The Principles of Physiology* (1834) and John Elliotson's *Human Physiology* (1835) as it was for such vulgarised publications as *The Book of Health* (1829), *The Express, or Every Man His Own Doctor* (1823), *The Physiology of Health* (1841) and *The Poor Man's Medical Guide in Emergency* (1823). The reason for such omission was spelled out by Henry Bickersteth in *Medical Hints* (1829). It was not the doctor's duty, he declared, to instruct laymen on the details of procreation, for such information might be then used to escape the punishment ordained by God for sexual misdemeanours:

> In female complaints some other questions are necessary; but it is not intended to extend these directions to them, nor to that disease which the Almighty has been pleased to inflict as a bitter scourge on the unlawful indulgence between the sexes.[10]

The attitude of the quacks towards sexuality was quite different. They did provide some crude analysis of the functioning of the reproductive system, but their main purpose was, of course, not to give an accurate account of human physiology. Their purpose was to terrorise the male public, with tales of the horrible consequences of sexual excesses, into the purchase of restorative cordials and medications. Rather than assure the reader that there was knowledge available which could permit him to avoid illness, quacks claimed that only their 'secret' remedies could cure the 'nervous debility' into which all would eventually plunge. In a similar fashion, quacks attributed a whole range of female diseases to disruption of the menstrual cycle. A wide variety of 'French' or 'female pills' were guaranteed to cure a 'suppression of the menses'. The distributors of such medications, though they paraded their concern that their products be used in an attempt to terminate pregnancy, implied that they were abortifacients and no doubt many women purchased them for this reason.

What was the response of the medical profession to the public's interest in reproduction and in particular the possibility of controlling births? It is impossible to know what individual doctors told their patients in the privacy of their consulting rooms; this analysis must therefore be confined to prescriptive medical literature.[11] Even this is scarce for the first half of the nineteenth century, and relatively few medical men made allusions to actual birth control practices or 'precautions'. In *Observations on the Mortality and Physical Management of Children* (1827) John Roberton the Elder simply acknowledged that 'Since the publication of Malthus' profound work on population many absurd, and some criminal, notions have been promulgated on the subject of CHECKS to the increase of mankind, most of them originating in a misapprehension of the opinion of this writer'.[12] Doctors, however, could not ignore the public's attempt to regulate births. The common occurrence of abortion was frequently noted in the medical press.[13] 'In some of the manufacturing districts', wrote a contributor to the *Cottage Physician,* 'the use of large doses of Epsom or Glauber's salts to procure abortion, is understood to be very common. . .'[14] If one is to believe the editor of Buchan's *Domestic Medicine,* abortionists were by 1827 using the press to advertise both their products and services: 'I never heard without shuddering any advertisement of temporary retreats, or pretended accommodations for pregnant ladies. . .'[15] The low illegitimacy rate of the factory towns of Lancashire was frequently attributed to working women's recourse to abortifacients. As W.R. Greg observed: 'The deduction we draw is also materially confirmed by the practice, which it is painful to state, is far from uncommon among the abandoned females of these districts of destroying prematurely the fruit and evidence of their guilt.'[16] Dr Robert Venables was so concerned that even those references to therapeutic abortions contained in erudite medical texts would'. . . circulate among the vulgar and less-informed classes of society . . .' via the popular press that he refrained from dealing with the topic in print.[17]

The factory reports of 1831 and 1833, moreover, revealed that doctors were aware of the circulation of birth control tracts in working-class districts. Dr James Blundell declared that'. . . where individuals are congregated as in the factories, I conceive that means preventive of impregnation are most likely to be generally known and practised by young persons'.[18] Dr Hunter referred to'. . . books or pamphlets, which are a disgrace to any age or country' being offered for sale in Leeds.[19] The doctors disagreed on the question whether such knowledge of contraception was actually put into practical use, but they were as one in expressing their disgust at the publication of this information.

A complete condemnation of birth control was finally provided in *The Philosophy of Marriage* (1837) by Dr Michael Ryan, who began the book by upbraiding his colleagues for their reticence on the subject: 'Are not the most revolting vices now unblushingly recommended as checks to population? and are not the most immoral works circulated and exposed in almost every bye-street through which we pass?'[20] Ryan then proceeded to condemn on medical grounds such 'checks' because the 'various abominable means' proposed to regulate births were not only immoral but '. . . were contrary to the dictates of nature'. He finally said openly what other medical observers would only allude to in their condemnation of birth control – namely that the availability of safe contraception would undermine the existing family structure:

> None can deny that, if young women in general were absolved from the fear of consequences, the great majority of them, unless the comparatively few who are strictly moral and highly educated, would rarely preserve their chastity; illicit amours would be common and seldom detected – seduction would be facilitated, and prostitution become almost universal, unless among the virtuous and small class, already accepted.[21]

In short the doctor saw his main duty as maintaining the existing moral code rather than as supplying medical information desired by a segment of the population.

The response of the medical profession to the birth control issue, however, was not simply negative. Some medical men in the first half of the nineteenth century recognised the need for family planning and saw that mere counsels of abstinence were insufficient. Dr Henry Oldham, lecturer on midwifery at Guy's Hospital, presumably expressed the feelings of many doctors: 'It constantly happens that cases come before us where either from disease of the uterus or pelvis, or sexual organs, or exhaustion from frequent abortions or protracted labours – that it would be most desirable to suspend for a time or altogether prevent pregnancy.'[22] There were now in fact effective means of preventing conception already available – the sheath, the douche, the sponge and coitus interuptus. Doctors would not, however, discuss any of these metnods, all of which they considered to be associated with prostitution and immorality. Thus during the mid-nineteenth century there was the curious situation of doctors, who saw the necessity of controlling conception, spurning reliable, well-established methods and devoting their attention to the discovery of 'natural' methods that would not be tainted by association with 'unnatural' acts. Dr Charles Loudon, for example, who had chaired the medical committee of the Factory Report of 1833 and heard evidence on the extent of abortion in the Midlands, attempted to prove in *The Equilibrium of*

Population and Sustenance Demonstrated (1836) that extended nursing could be used to limit a woman's fertility.[23] Greater interest was shown in the theory, advanced by the French physicians Pouchet and Raciborski in the late 1840s, that the calculation of a woman's ovulation cycle permitted the determination of 'safe' or sterile periods.[24] This rhythm method was for the moment to prove ineffective because the safe period was mistakenly judged to occur immediately after menstruation, but the appeal that it and the lactation method had for doctors was that both were 'natural' and medically approved.[25] Doctors who interested themselves in the question used these apparent advances in medical science to exalt the pretensions of the profession. While they extolled their methods, they thus continued to denigrate all other types of birth control as both morally and physically dangerous. This would even be true of Dr George Drysdale who in 1855 was to be the first doctor in England to write, albeit anonymously, in defence of contraception. However, while accepting the efficacy of the sponge, he attacked coitus interruptus as leading to 'sexual infeeblement and congestion' and the sheath for 'producing impotence in the man and disgust in both parties'.[26]

It would be misleading to leave the impression that the medical profession was actively debating the pros and cons of birth control in the first half of the nineteenth century. Its main response to the issue of 'artificial' means of contraception was almost total silence. Dr Ryan's *Philosophy of Marriage,* which condemned birth control, was in turn condemned by the *British and Foreign Medical Review* for even dealing with such an objectionable subject.[27] The writings of the birth control advocates were completely ignored by the British professional journals, while in America the *Boston Medical Journal* felt obliged to apologise for even noting the appearance of Knowlton's *Fruits of Philosophy*:

> We think, however, the less that is known about it (the book) by the public at large, the better it will be for the morals of the community; and it is only as the production of a medical man, and in a work read by medical men that we have thought it expedient to notice it.[28]

The official silence of the profession would be maintained for the greater part of the century.[29]

The silence of doctors was in fact the most eloquent expression of their hostility to the whole issue of birth control. Such hostility reflected, of course, the contemporary attitudes of respectable society. It has, moreover, to be recalled that the social standing of the profession was in the very process of being established; its members were accordingly sensitive to the dangers of association with disreputable doctrines. Gynaecologists and obstetricians, who were seeking to convince the public that '. . . one sex only is qualified by education and powers of mind to investigate what the other sex has alone to suffer',[30] were, not surprisingly, the most cautious. Since the nature of their speciality left them open to the charge of violating public decency, they were all the more adamant in their defence of traditional moral norms.[31] In Dr E.J. Tilt's words:

> I shall remind the reader that a profession which has the confidence of women holds in its hands the fate of society. . . (it has the) power, not only for the curing of disease, and the maintenance of individual health, but also for imparting a healthy tone to society, and for the healing of its wounds.[32]

If the doctor had defended contraception he would have risked his reputation; by defending traditional morality with new scientific arguments he assumed the position previously monopolised by the priest — defender of public virtue. The medical profession was to take a jaundiced view of all health reforms and home cures; its disavowal of birth control was all the more understandable inasmuch as it irritated both its moral and professional susceptibilities.[33]

The activities of the advocates of birth control take on increased significance when placed in this context. On the one hand quacks were exploiting the public's ignorance in sexual matters; on the other the medical profession was refusing to recognise birth control as a medical question with which it should involve itself.

The first guarded references to the need for birth control were contained in the writings of the Utilitarians, but widespread interest in the question was stimulated only after the distribution in 1823 by Francis Place of handbills explaining in detail methods of contraception.[34] William Thompson, the communitarian theorist provided an extended moral and economic argument for such practices in *An Enquiry into the Principles of the Distribution of Wealth* (1824) and in *Practical Directions for the Speedy and Economical Establishment of Communities* (1830). The first book devoted to the subject of contraception was Richard Carlile's *Every Woman's Book* (1826).[35] Carlile described the techniques mentioned by Place — the sponge, the sheath and withdrawal. The same methods were recommended by Robert Dale Owen in *Moral Physiology* (1831) and Charles Knowlton, who added information on the douche, in *Fruits of Philosophy* (1832).[36]

The medical arguments that the birth controllers advanced in their defence of contraception were quite straightforward. They asserted that they were only responding to a situation to which doctors had turned a blind eye:

> All states of pain are evil: all states of pleasure are good. The greater amount of animal life is a state of pain, and the duty of humanity, virtue or what is called morality, is to lessen the amount of pain; and the principle of preventing painful conceptions is a positive good to society.[37]

The working class was already using injurious means in an attempt to regulate births, and was thereby making known its need for reliable methods. To supply such knowledge would result in the diminution of abortion and infanticide. It would spare women unwanted pregnancies, attendant illnesses, and the dangers of miscarriage. Marriages would no longer have to be postponed for financial reasons, and as a result masturbation, prostitution and similar unhealthy substitutes for legitimate intercourse would disappear. The married would be more faithful and youth more chaste. Women would no longer be viewed as simple propagators of the species but as men's helpmates. The plight of orphans, bastards, and women dying in labour or during induced abortions could, claimed the birth controllers, all be avoided.[38]

With the appearance of the birth control tracts the artisan interested in the question of reproduction finally had something to refer to in addition to *Aristotle's Works* and the quacks' terrifying handbills. The nineteenth-century doctors might condemn the charlatan's treatises on sexuality, but they were loath to provide an alternative. It was left to the birth controllers both to supply the public with accurate information and to combat as best they could popular prejudices. One could thus by the 1830s find in the penny press, alongside advertisements for Solomon's Cordial Balm of Gilead and Dr H's Golden Anti-Venereal Pills, announcements on the sale of Owen's *Moral Physiology* and Knowlton's *Fruits of Philosophy.* [39] The birth control literature, however, was condemned by the medical profession while, in the words of Knowlton, '. . .other works of like purpose, as well as that dirty useless thing called *Aristotle* are publicly sold with impunity'.[40]

The relationship between the birth controllers and the medical profession was not a simple one. The birth controllers, on the one hand sought to give the impression that their efforts received medical support. Francis Place claimed in his handbills that the methods he described were recommended by 'eminent physicians' and 'first-rate accoucheurs'.[41] According to Robert Dale Owen's *Moral Physiology,* English and French doctors agreed that contraception could be practised '. . .without any injury to health'.[42] Richard Carlile stated that '. . .where a state of health will not justify a pregnancy, it is common, in London for the physician to recommend the means of prevention, for it is well understood, that abstinence and domestic happiness cannot co-exist'.[43] The birth controllers, on the other hand, maintained that doctors had no intention of spreading contraceptive information. They implied that doctors had access to knowledge which they were limiting to an elite. Indeed the idea that the lower classes should take advantage of methods hitherto monopolised by the wealthy was repeatedly touched on in the birth control tracts. Carlile noted that 'The remedy has long been known in this country and to the aristocracy in particular, who are always in search of benefits which they can particularly hold, and be distinct from the body of the labouring people.'[44] In short the birth controllers were appealing to the artisans' suspicion of their 'betters' and, in particular, the suspicion that the medical profession was drawing benefits from the ignorance of the people.[45]

The extent to which the birth controllers themselves viewed the profession with suspicion was a function of their attitudes towards social reform. Place, a believer in *Laissez-faire* made it clear in his own life that he had more confidence in his own bleeding techniques and cold water treatments than in medical prescriptions, but at the same time he made no public criticism of doctors.[46] Charles Knowlton, a medical man himself, attacked his profession's failure to deal with the crucial question of procreation: 'In books, pamphlets, journals, etc., they have laid much before the public representing eating, drinking, bathing, lacing, air, exercises, etc., but have passed by this still more important subject now before us, giving only here and there some faint allusion to it.'[47]

Knowlton sought to take information to the people not only through his writings but also in 'A Course of Physiological Lectures as Connected with Moral Philosophy' at Frances Wright's Hall of Science in New York.[48] For Carlile, a crusader for political reform, the medical profession's attempt to monopolise certain types of knowledge represented yet another aspect of 'Old Corruption', and he accordingly labelled doctors '. . .as wicked a set of imposters as priests'.[49] It was the writings of the communitarians, William Thompson and Robert Dale Owen, however, which contained the most thorough denunciation of organised medicine. For Thompson most diseases were the simple consequence of '. . .imprudence, intemperance, and distraction of other vices'.[50] In the existing competitive society the doctor benefited from the spread of disease and had no interest in the sort of preventive medicine which birth control represented:

> Competition calls into being a set of men who necessarily trade in the curing of wounds and diseases. The more wounds and diseases, if accompanied with the ability of paying for the cure, the better for this trade, as the greater the demand for cottons and silks the better for the manufacturers of these articles. . .It is moreover no part of their (the doctors) profession, as it has been no part of their study, to preserve health to the healthy; it is on the contrary their vulgar interest, as forming one of the trades of competition, that the healthy should become diseased.[51]

Only in a society of 'Mutual Cooperation' would the citizen find his good health the subject of the interest of his fellows.[52] In the reformed society each would be taught '. . .what every human being ought to know, the physiology. . .of the human frame and the laws of health'.[53] The sexual passions would at last be understood by all and be permitted to '. . .find their level of gentle and healthful gratification and contentment: and when all possible consequential evils, such as an injurious increase in numbers or abstraction of time from useful employments, are by appropriate regulations, guarded against, all the evils now arising from the misdirection of the passions would be avoided'.[54]

Owen followed very much the same line of reasoning as Thompson:

> But, however desirable for the masses of mankind that they should be taught how to retain the first of blessings, health; and that they should further be taught how to regain it, when lost; – it is *not* the interest of the physician. It is not his interest that his neighbours should know anything about their own bodies; it is not his interest that they should be taught how to retain their health, nor how to arrest an incipient malady by some simple remedy. Other men's ignorance is his gain. Their follies fill his purse. If they were educated as common sense dictates, he would be a poorer man. . . However beneficial, therefore, it might be, that we should know our own diseases and learn to prevent and cure them, we must not

> expect that physicians, as a class, will take much pains to destroy their own avocation. We must not expect them to tell us (however well they know it) that we are the best judges of our own sensations; that we can detect symptoms in ourselves that are hidden from them; that we have the most experience in our own constitutions; and that, thus, *even with an inferior knowledge of medical science,* we can prescribe much more readily and rationally for ourselves, than any other person can for us. We must not expect that physicians will risk at once their reputations and their fortunes, in order to tell us, that if we are but rational and practical physiologists, we should regret the morality which now prevails, as unnatural, and productive of suffering and disease; nor can we require that physicians should labour zealously to promote temperance and thus to prevent diseases. All this it were unreasonable to expect, because men do not like to ruin themselves, nor even to diminish their own earnings.[55]

Turning specifically to the question of sexuality, Owen declared that if one found an 'honest and enlightened physician' he would tell you,

> . . . of the prudish severity with which society dooms one sex to unnatural restraints, and of the temporising injustice with which she winks at the scarcely-veiled libertinism of the other. . .Ask him what *he* thinks of orthodox morality in itself and he will tell you, that *as a physiologist,* he disapproves and condemns it. But as a physician he profits by it. . .[56]

The birth controllers thus differed on the extent to which they believed social reform had to be pushed if disease was to be eradicated. Radicals such as Carlile and Place, whose political programmes were restricted to attacks on privilege, simply called for 'free trade' in medical knowledge. Socialists such as Owen and Thompson, who were sketching out plans for cooperative societies, seemed to be suggesting that in the future each man would be his own physician and the medical profession would wither away.[57] But all were agreed on the basic point that illness was largely a consequence of ignorance that could be overcome by medical self-help. In particular, the unnecessary sufferings of women in undesired pregnancies and the maladies of children of over-large families were declared to be a result of a lack of contraceptive knowledge.

Thus if the early birth control movement is looked at as a self-help medical movement, it becomes quite obvious why its advocates should have been hostile to the medical profession and why, in turn, physicians should have opposed contraception on professional as well as moral grounds. Doctors were trying to educate the nineteenth-century layman so as to instil in him a 'faith' in medicine. Their line of argument was well represented by Dr John Conolly who began *The Physician* with this comment:

> Unlike the common books of popular medicine, so eagerly purchased by the poorer as well as richer classes of readers, this publication is not meant to supersede an application of the sick to persons competent to cure them, but to show them that it is only in such persons that they can safely trust.[58]

The sponsors of the self-help medical movements were approaching the problem from the opposite angle; their goal was to instil in the layman a faith in himself and his ability to control his own life. Both groups sought to conquer disease; one believed it could be accomplished by reforming a profession – the other believed it required reforming a society.

Notes

1. On the history of birth control see Norman E. Himes, *A Medical History of Contraception,* Baltimore, 1936; J.A. Field, *Essays on Population,* Chicago, 1931; J.A. Banks, *Prosperity and Parenthood: A Study of Family Planning Among the Victorian Middle Classes,* London, 1954, and F.H. Amphlett Micklewright, 'The Rise and Fall of English Neo-Malthusianism', *Population Studies, 15,* 1961-2, 32-51.
2. Richard H. Shryock, *The Development of Modern Medicine,* London, 1948, p. 205 ff., and Brian Harrison, *Drink and the Victorians,* London, 1971, p. 185.
3. Michael Ryan, *Philosophy of Marriage,* London, 1837, p. 6.
4. See the essay by Janet Blackman, in this present volume, and also Otho T. Beall, '*Aristotle's Masterpiece* in America: A Landmark in the Folklore of Medicine', *William and Mary Quarterly, 20,* 1963, 207-22.
5. *The Works of Aristotle: His Complete Masterpiece,* London, 1772, p. 37.
6. See for example *Conjugal Love Reveal'd. . .Done from the French of Monsieur Vennette,* London, 1720; J. Ingle, *Pocket Companion to Culpeper's Herbal or English Physician,* London, 1820; (Author) Reid, *The Pleasures of Matrimony,* Glasgow, 1840, and E. Ward, *Female Policy Detected,* Glasgow, 1835. For poetical treatments see *Kick Him Jenny,* London, 1734, and John Armstrong, *The Oeconomy of Love,* London, 1739.
7. *Medical Times,* 28 September 1839, 6. See also John Corry, *The Detector of Quackery,* London, 1802; James Parkinson, *The Villager's Friend and Physician,* London, 1800, pp. 79-80; J.C. Feldman, *Quacks and*

Quackery Unmasked, London, 1842; *Monthly Gazette of Health*, *7*, 1822, 786; *Lancet*, 1842, *ii*, 781, and *Quarterly Review*, *141*, 1842-3, 83-105.

8. *Lancet*, 1851, *i*, 72-3.
9. Andrew Ure, *The Philosophy of Manufacturers*, London, 1835, p. 386. See also James Phillips Kay, *The Moral and Physical Condition of the Working Classes*, London, 1832, p. 65 ff.; Joseph Adshead, *Distress in Manchester: Evidence of the State of the Labouring Classes in 1840-1842*, London, 1842, p. 50; and Friedrich Engels, *The Condition of the Working Class in England in 1844*, London, 1950 edn., p. 104.
10. Henry Bickersteth, *Medical Hints*, London, 1829. For doctors' jealousy of the quacks' success in exploiting the concern with venereal complaints see Robert John Thornton, *The Medical Guardian of Youth*, London, 1816, pp. 71-2 and 86-7; James Thorn, *An Attempt to Simplify the Treatment of Sexual Diseases* London, 1831, p. 11 and Michael Ryan, *A Manual of Midwifery*, 3rd edn., London 1831, p. 377.
11. For an overview see John Peel, 'Contraception and the Medical Profession', *Population Studies*, *18*, 1964-5, 133-46.
12. John Roberton the Elder, *Observations on the Mortality and Physical Management of Children*, London, 1827, p. 5. See also John Wade, *History of the Middle and Working Classes*, London, 1833, p. 337.
13. See for example the *Lancet* from 1827 onwards.
14. *The Cottage Physician*, London, 1825, p. 59. The contemporary literature also refers to the use of knitting needles, savine and ergot of rye to precipitate abortions.
15. William Buchan, *Domestic Medicine or, the Family Physician*, London, 1827 edn., p. viii.
16. W.R. Greg, *An Inquiry into the State of the Manufacturing Population* London, 1831, p. 25. See also Edward Lytton Bulwer, *England and the English*, London, 1833, vol. I, p. 204; P. Gaskell, *The Manufacturing Population of England*, London, 1833, p. 85; William Dodd, *The Factory System Illustrated*, London, 1842, p. 26, and Lord Ashley's proposed amendment on 15 March 1844 during the debate on the Factory Bill, *Hansard's Parliamentary Debates*, third series, *73*, 1844, col. *1093*. On the claim that infanticide was being practised in working districts see Lyon Playfair, *Report on the State of Large Towns in Lancashire*, London, 1845, p. 128 ff., and James Simpson, *A Probationary Essay on Infanticide*, Edinburgh, 1825.
17. *London Medical Gazette*, 10 September 1831, 777-8.
18. 'Committee on the Factories' Bill', *Parliamentary Papers*, *XV*, 1831-2.
19. 'Dr. Loudon's Medical Report', *Parliamentary Papers*, *XXI*, 1833.
20. Ryan (1837), *op. cit.*, p. 6.
21. *Ibid.*, p. 10.
22. Henry Oldham, 'Clinical Lecture on the Induction of Abortion in a Case of Contracted Vagina from Cicatrisation', *London Medical Gazette*, *9*, 1849, 48.
23. See also Charles Loudon, *Solution du Probleme de la Population et de la Subsistence*, Paris, 1842; T. Laycock, 'On the Influence of Lactation in Preventing the Recurrence of Pregnancy', *Dublin Medical Press*, no. 199, 1842, 263-4, and John Roberton the Younger, *Essays and Notes on the Physiology and Diseases of Women and on Practical Midwifery*, London, 1851.
24. For an account of French theories of ovulation see Angus McLaren, 'Doctor in the House: Medicine and Private Morality in France, 1800-1850', *Feminist Studies*, *2*, 1975, 39-54. On the English response see

Oldham, *op. cit;* Charles Ritchie, 'On General Disease', *Edinburgh Medical and Surgical Journal, 75,* 1851, 31 ff., and James Whitehead, *On the Causes and Treatment of Abortion and Sterility,* London, 1847, p. 30.

25. For the popularisation of the 'rhythm method' see Edward Ruddock, *Affections of Females,* London, 1861 and his *The Common Diseases of Women,* 6th edn., London 1888; G.H. Napheys, *The Physical Life of Women,* Philadelphia, 1869, and Anon., *Valuable Hints to Fathers Having Increasing Families but Limited Incomes,* London, 1866.
26. George Drysdale, *The Elements of Social Science,* London, 1867, p. 349. The first anonymous edition of 1855 was entitled *Physical, Sexual and Natural Religion.*
27. *British and Foreign Medical Review, 5,* 1838, 443-6.
28. *Boston Medical Journal, 27,* 1843, 256.
29. On the reluctance of doctors to say anything about sex see S. Mason, *The Philosophy of Female Health,* London, 1845, p. 1 ff., and John Pocock Holmes, *Popular Observations on Diseases Incident to Females,* London, 1831, p. vi.
30. Edward J. Tilt, *On Diseases of Women and Ovarian Inflammation,* London, 1853, p. 9. For advice to women on how they should discuss their problems with the physician see A. Lady (E.W. Farrar), *The Young Lady's Friend,* London, 1837, p. 53, and Holmes, *op. cit.,* p. 24.
31. On the old suspicion of obstetricians see P. Thicknesse, *Man Midwifery Analysed and the Tendency of that Practice Detected and Exposed,* London, 1764, and his *The Danger and Immodesty of the Present Custom of Unnecessarily Employing Men-Midwives,* London, 1772; J. Blunt, *Man-Midwifery Dissected,* London, 1793, and M. Adams, *Man-Midwifery Exposed,* London, 1830.
32. Edward J. Tilt, *On the Preservation of the Health of Women at the Critical Periods of Life,* London, 1851, p. 41.
33. On the continuing hostility of the profession see the *British Medical Journal,* 1868, *ii,* 113 and John W. Taylor, *On the Diminishing Birth Rate* London, 1904.
34. On Place's role see the notes and introduction of Norman E. Himes to Francis Place, *Illustrations and Proofs of Principle of Population,* 2nd edn., London, 1930, and G.J. Holyoake, *Sixty Years of an Agitator's Life,* London, 1900, vol. I, p. 126 ff.
35. It first appeared as *What is Love?* in Carlile's *Republican,* 6 May 1825 and was then later brought out as a pamphlet in February 1826. Eight editions were produced by 1828.
36. Norman E. Himes, 'Charles Knowlton's Revolutionary Influence on the English Birth Rate', *New England Journal of Medicine, 199,* 1928, 461-5.
37. Carlile, *Every Women's Book,* London, 1838, p. 37. It should be recalled that some doctors even considered the administering of anaesthetics to women in labour as a violation of the biblical injunction 'In sorrow shall she bring forth'. See J.Y. Simpson, *Answer to Religious Objections Advanced Against the Employment of Anaesthetic Agents in Midwifery and Surgery,* Edinburgh, 1847.
38. Carlile (1838), *op. cit.,* pp. 19 and 23-4; Robert Dale Owen, *Moral Physiology,* New York, 1831, pp. 35-6; and Charles Knowlton, *Fruits of Philosophy,* London, 1841 edn., pp. 37 and 40.
39. See for example the *Examiner, Crisis, Poor Man's Guardian, Destructive, Working Man's Friend and Political Magazine,* and *Fly.*
40. Boston *Investigator,* 11 January 1833.
41. See also Place, *op. cit.,* p. 324.
42. Owen, *op. cit.,* p. 60.

43. T. Carlile, *The Lion*, 3 October 1828.
44. *Ibid.*
45. On the extent of the working-class suspicion of physicians which manifested itself at the time of the 1832 cholera epidemic see the *Poor Man's Guardian*, 25 February and 8 September 1832; *The Cosmopolite*, 8 September 1832; Henry Gaulter, *The Origins and Progress of the Malignant Cholera in Manchester*, London 1833, pp. 137-8; James Simpson, *Necessity of Popular Education as a National Object*, Boston, 1834, p. 23, and Mary Thale (ed.), *The Autobiography of Francis Place, 1771-1854*, London, 1972, *passim.*
47. Knowlton, *op. cit.*, p. 37.
48. An American defender of Knowlton wrote: 'He has made the knowledge too cheap; and that is not the worst of it, he has permitted common people, people who can be benefitted by the knowledge to have access to it.' *Boston Investigator*, 15 February 1833.
49. *The Republican*, 11 March 1825. See also the attack on doctors made by Carlile's wife, Eliza Sharples, in *Isis*, 2 June 1832.
50. William Thompson, *Appeal to One Half of the Human Race, Women, Against the Pretensions of the Other Half, Men*, London, 1825, p. 142.
51. William Thomson, *Practical Directions for the Speedy and Economical Establishment of Communities*, London, 1830, p. 195.
52. William Thompson, *Labour Rewarded: The Claims of Labour and Capital Conciliated*, London, 1827, p. 67.
53. William Thompson, *An Inquiry into the Principles of the Distribution of Wealth*, London, 1824, p. 339.
54. Thompson (1830), *op. cit.*, pp. 200-1.
55. *Free Inquirer*, 18 February 1829.
56. *Ibid.* See also Robert Dale Owen, *Situations: Lawyers-Clergy-Physicians-Men and Women*, London, 1840 and Joel Pinny, *An Exposure of the Causes of the Present Deteriorated Condition of Health*, London, 1830, p. 165.
57. Owen and Thompson were the only socialists to argue in favour of contraception, but it should be noted that all the communitarians of the 1830s were sympathetic to the less controversial forms of fringe medicine such as vegetarianism, teetotalism, and fresh air and cold water treatments. See J.F.C. Harrison, *Robert Owen and the Owenties in Britain and America*, London, 1969, p. 179.
58. John Conolly, *The Physician*, London, 1832, p. 9.

4 DOCTORS AND WOMEN IN NINETEENTH-CENTURY SOCIETY: SEXUALITY AND ROLE

Jean L'Esperance

In recent years, and following promptings from the contemporary women's movement, a whole host of male-dominated viewpoints have been challenged. In this context ideas of the medical profession, and particularly its treatment of women, are being critically re-examined.[1] Socio-historical studies of nineteenth-century scientific and medical attitudes are revealing that doctors used new scientific discoveries to validate conventional ideas about femininity and woman's sexuality, and woman's role in society. New techniques in gynaecological surgery, and new scientific discoveries, such as the place of ovulation in the menstrual cycle, were used to reinforce all the existing assumptions about femininity which were prevalent in nineteenth-century culture.[2] This essay examines several important medical works, and their statement of commonly accepted views regarding the nature of male and female sexuality, and attempts to chart some of the areas in which women themselves rejected the man-made stereotype and challenged the growing power and status of the predominantly male medical profession.

The essay begins with a comment on the existence and role of a 'double standard' for sexual behaviour – a belief made possible by an apparent acceptance by both sexes of woman's passive and 'pure' role. Treatises on sexuality assumed a male dominance and made little reference to woman's sexuality. The ideas of Acton, Tissot, Lallemand and Drysdale are briefly described. As changes in both scientific knowledge and in social structure (and in this context, particularly woman's role) take place, so predominant and sterotyped views come to be challenged. How and why did women accept the male viewpoint regarding sexuality? A partial erosion of this view, which had become institutionalised in society, is considered in relation to a growing recognition afforded to the ideas of such pioneers and reformers as Elizabeth Garrett Anderson, Elizabeth Blackwell and Josephine Butler. Role relationships and conflicts, involving *inter alia* occupation and sex, were clearly undergoing change: thus in the final section of the essay there follow brief references to the increasing demand for women doctors, and to the involvement of women both in campaigns to enhance the status of nursing and midwifery, and also in 'anti-medical' movements.

During the early part of the nineteenth century, the essential core of the conventional attitude towards sexual behaviour was a widespread conviction that social order rested upon the 'double standard' – that is, the belief that there was one moral code of sexual behaviour for men, and another for women.[3] Despite living in a nominally Christian society which subscribed to a belief in strict continence outside of marriage for both sexes, Jonathan Dymond, when he published his treatise on *Principles of Morality* in 1829, discovered that there was no greater disparity between the assessment of wickedness according to both the moral law and public opinion than in regard to male unchastity. The figure of twenty was used in his compilation to indicate both 'the highest degree of reprobation in the Moral Law', and the 'highest offence according to popular opinion':

	Moral Law	*Public Opinion*
Murder	20	20
Human destruction under other names	18	0
Unchastity, if of women	18	18
Unchastity, if of men	18	2

Commenting on the latter difference, Dymond remarked that it was 'discordant to excess'.[4]

Public disapproval of a woman who had 'fallen' from respectability by 'fast' behaviour, known or open indulgence in extra-marital sex, or the bearing of an illegitimate child, was concretely expressed by making her a social outcast.[5] Even if the origins of this view can be traced back to the seventeenth century, mid-nineteenth-century Britain saw the high water mark of a belief in the 'double standard' and the first concerted revolt against it by women. It was not as an expression of pure hostility or dislike that women were treated more harshly than men. Their sexual lapses were more severely treated simply because they were considered to be by nature purer and finer than the male sex. Any fall from a high standard of behaviour was more culpable, since it was 'unnatural' and depraved. The sexual passivity and nullity of the truly 'womanly' woman was judged to be vitally important for the sexual economy of the male.[6]

The mid-nineteenth century was a significant period in the development of the medical profession. It witnessed the efforts by Simon to evolve a network of state medicine, and those of a group of medical reformers to establish professional standards, and a sound educational basis for the profession.[7] As a whole, however, the profession still felt a certain insecurity, for the public health legislation in the middle years of the century had at times been passed in spite of medical opposition. Indeed the vital question, 'is a medical man a gentleman?' was often raised among neutral observers of the Victorian social scene.[8] This led many doctors to adopt a committed stance and to make strong pronouncements on a wide range of social problems on which they were not necessarily experts: 'The demonstrations achieved by medical science have needed and still need to be pressed upon public men with incessant energy, in order to effect the necessary reforms.'[9] Increasing demand for medical care on the part of the middle classes, combined with a growing perception of medical attention as a status symbol by those below, also added to the social power of the doctor. This power was, doctors believed, to be used to bolster the best interests of society. When Lord Amberley called on the profession to discover non-injurious forms of contraception, the *Medical Times and Gazette* indignantly remarked:

> . . . for the honour of our Profession for the truest and best interests of our country, and in the name of public decency and domestic purity, we feel it to be our duty to give no uncertain note on this question, and to protest in the most solemn manner as responsible to a higher power, against the possibility of infringing natural laws without entailing upon ourselves sundry diseases and divers kinds of death.[10]

Medical ideas about male sexuality were permeated by the profound anxiety which any sexual act aroused in Mid-Victorian society. For men, the loss of sperm, through intercourse or any other activity, was a dangerous and debilitating act. Sperm represented 'the concentrated powers of a man's perfected being' and loss of sperm meant loss of that energy necessary for the competitive struggle which typified middle-class life.[11] The secretion of sperm was the vital component of that feeling of virility 'necessary to give a man that consciousness of his dignity, of his character as head and ruler, and of his importance, which is absolutely essential to the well-being of the family, and through it, of society itself'.[12] Loss of sperm, it was thought, was particularly dangerous in adolescence, for it might drain away the energy needed to develop the mature man. In keeping with this philosophy there was published from the 1830s onwards a constant stream of manuals and handbooks which tried to help young men avoid all incontinence, and especially that major cause of it, masturbation.[13] This habit was 'one of the most serious and frequent causes of disease in youth'. The majority of the worst causes of seminal weakness which doctors saw were, it was believed, undoubtedly due to this habit – indeed masturbation was adjudged to cause more excitement than sexual intercourse, since it was 'more frequently repeated, and consequently more injurious to health and more productive of disease'.[14] As described by William Acton, the adolescent who indulged in this practice was hardly an appealing figure:

> The frame is stunted and weak, the muscles undeveloped, the eye is sunken and heavy, the complexion is sallow, pasty or covered with spots of acne, the hands are damp and cold, and the skin moist. The boy shuns the society of others, creeps about alone, joins with repugnance in the amusements of his schoolfellows. He cannot look anyone in the face, and becomes careless in dress and uncleanly in person. His intellect is often of the lowest class, and if his evil habits are persisted in, he may end in becoming a drivelling idiot or a peevish valetudinarian.[15]

Not only was masturbation thought to be the cause of much ill-health: it was felt it could also lead to homosexuality.[16] Contemporary writers were well aware of the prevalence of homosexual practices among men in prison, on board ship and in penal colonies, and they deprecated its moral and physical results even more than those of masturbation.[17] In the eighteenth century it was believed that masturbation was productive of disease. The origins of this idea seem to spring from two sources, the second being more influential than the first. The first was the pamphlet, *Onania: or the Heinous Sin of Self-Pollution and All its Frightful Consequences in Both Sexes Consider'd,* first published in 1710. The anonymous author listed as results of the practice 'stranguries, priapisms and gonorrhoeas, thin and waterish seed, fainting fits and epilepsies, consumptions, loss of erections and premature ejaculation, consumption and infertility'. Women who indulged in the habit were, in addition, subject to imbecility, leucorrhea, hysteric fits and barrenness, while the children of habitual masturbators would be 'a Misery to themselves, a dishonour to Human Race (sic), and a Scandal to their Parents'.[18] The pamphlet's effectiveness can be gauged from the many editions published, and the numerous letters from grateful readers printed in subsequent editions. The second and possibly real basis for the widespread nineteenth-century fear of masturbation, however, seems to have been an influential work by the Swiss physician, Samuel Tissot. His *Tentamen de Morbis ex Manustruprat-ione,* written in 1758 and subsequently translated by the author in 1760 as *L'Onanisme, ou dissertation physique sur les maladies produites par la masturbation,* was widely circulated, being soon further translated into English (in 1766 by A. Hume), German and Italian. Tissot, while agreeing with the *Onania* about the consequences of masturbation, gave the belief a scientific basis, when he explained that the practice involved an excessive and unnatural loss of 'la liqueur seminale' and that the nervous energy was drained from the brain by the act, leaving a permanent scar. The orgasm, Tissot explained, was a form of compulsive spasm which upset the body's carefully balanced mechanism. He cited other respected eighteenth-century physicians, such as Hoffman and Boerhaave, who also predicted dire injurious consequences from loss of semen, either through masturbation or nocturnal emissions. Although sections of the medical professions had, by the beginning of the nineteenth century, refuted these ideas, Tissot was still accepted at the popular level, and by a number of reputable practitioners such as William Acton. Tissot's theories gained a new lease of life in the early nineteenth century by the discovery of the disease 'spermatorrhoea' or involuntary seminal loss, often brought on, or aggravated by persistent masturbation.

The most influential writer on this affliction was Lallemand, whose *Des Pertes Seminales* (translated as *On Involuntary Seminal Discharges*) was widely read. 'I have collected', he wrote, 'within thirteen or fourteen years, more than one hundred and fifty cases of involuntary seminal losses, grave enough to produce serious derangement of health, and even to cause death.'[19] His subjects had often indulged in excessive excitation of the genital parts, either through coition or masturbation. Every abundant seminal evacuation through 'diurnal or nocturnal pollutions' constituted spermatorrhoea, even though they might have taken place without erection and entirely without pleasure. Lallemand, unlike his English and American disciples, who preferred to prescribe cold sponge baths and gymnastic exercises, often recommended intercourse as a cure for spermatorrhoea. His medical vocabulary, however, was full of moral homilies, and he urged his fellow doctors to study and tackle 'a disease that degrades man, poisons the happiness of his best days and ravages society'.

Support for Lallemand came from William Acton, the leading venereologist of his day, whose *The Functions and Disorders of the Reproductive Organs in Childhood, in Youth, in Adult Age, and in Advanced Life, considered in their Physiological, Social and Moral Relations* was written in a 'calm and philosophic spirit' to tell the truth about the disease which had caused so much suffering to the male sex. *The Functions and Disorders* was inappropriately titled since, apart from two passages, it dealt with only *male* reproductive organs, whose use should be avoided as much as possible. Sexual activity, Acton believed, was overwhelmingly debilitating – 'all men require restraint, not excitement'.[20] Careful management, in childhood especially, was needed:

> . . . the premature development of the sexual inclination is not alone repugnant to all we associate with the term childhood, but is also fraught with danger to his dawning manhood. Extreme youth should be attended by complete repose of the generative functions, unbroken by anything like even a desire for their enjoyment.[21]

Acton considered that if sexual precocity were observed in the child, it could often be explained as the result of inheritance from parents who had indulged in sexual excess. Masturbation often started in boyhood from mere curiosity, and had to be most carefully avoided; although the bad effect came at this early age from nervous excitement rather than from loss of semen, a child could still seriously impair his health. 'He should be taught', advised Acton, 'to look upon masturbation as a cowardly, selfish, debasing habit and one which should preclude those who practice it from associating with boys of proper spirit.'[22] Learning to resist the temptation to masturbate was in itself, for the middle-class boy, a valuable educational experience: '. . . artificial stimulus brings the upper classes and civilised societies, under a probation which sifts them justly, and provides for the deterioration and downfall of those who do not stand the test'.[23]

With the onset of puberty, and the development of sexual desire, even greater care had to be taken to train the boy to continence, defined by Acton as 'voluntary and entire abstinence from sexual indulgence in any form'. Life, he explained, should be spent in work, laying the foundations of success in life, and no man should think of marriage until he had established himself. Marriage itself, even though providing the only safe sexual outlet, could be dangerous to male health, possibly leading to marital excess, which had the same weakening effects as other sexual activities. The rest of Acton's book dealt with life after fifty and when sexual activity of any kind should, he averred, be completely avoided if a healthy old age was to be enjoyed.

Reviews in the medical press of *The Functions and Disorders. . .* showed clearly that Acton's views were not considered to be exaggerated: 'We think Mr. Acton has done good service to society by grappling manfully with sexual vices and we trust that others, whose position as men of science and teachers enable them to speak with authority, will assist in combating and arresting the evils which it entails . . .'[24] Spermatorrhoea was taken seriously even by doctors who denounced 'the horrors of the Manly Vigour School and spermatorrhoea quacks'. John Laws Milton, in a series of articles reprinted from the *Lancet,* cited and criticised the works of Lalemand and Acton – and others such as Phillips, Curling and Russell. He claimed that spermatorrhoea was 'a disease *per se',* and believed that incontinence could induce it.[25]

George Drysdale, who under the pseudonym 'a Graduate of Medicine', published the immensely popular *The Elements of Social Science, or Physical, Social and Natural Religion,* also warned against masturbation and spermatorrhoea, even though his attitude to sexual activity was completely opposed to that of Acton. Drysdale believed that the genitals would wither away if they were not exercised, and also that sexual abstinence was one of the chief causes of disease in men and women. Masturbation, he claimed, was one of the most frequent causes of disease in youth and 'the majority of the worst cases of seminal weakness are owing to this cause'.[26] He continued:

> It is a disgrace to medicine and mankind that so important a class of diseases, and those of the genital organs, have become a trade and speculation of unscientific men, because forsooth they are looked upon unfavourably by society, and even by some of our own proofession. Until this class of diseases receive due respect from all, and till no greater blame attach to them than to any other violation of natural laws and consequent disease, so long shall we be disgusted by the degrading advertisement of 'silent friends', 'cures for certain diseases' etc., in reading which one's breast glows with indignation and sorrow.[27]

Drysdale's suggested cure for masturbation, however, was not continence but natural sexual intercourse.

In the latter half of the nineteenth-century masturbation theories underwent a change; the emphasis shifted from the physical to the mental consequences of spermatic loss. Fielding Blandford, in *Insanity and its Treatment* (1871), claimed that the brain underwent permanent damage from the habit of masturbation.[28] It was to save their endangered minds, not their morals, that Isaac Baker Brown excised the clitoris of his female patients in the London Surgical Home.[29]

Literature on masturbation and spermatorrhoea used 'science' and growing medical knowledge to reinforce a widespread network of beliefs about the nature of male sexuality – beliefs which were largely unexamined and questioned, and in which the woman had an indispensable but totally secondary role. She existed to satisfy man's sexual and emotional needs, and bear children. Although man's sexual desires could be very strong, they could be controlled by the mind, if the recommendations of Acton and his colleagues were followed. By contrast, it has been argued, women were completely at the mercy of their biology.[30]

The enforcement of the 'double standard' was made possible by widespread acceptance among both sexes of the woman's essentially passive, pure nature. She was a naturally virtuous being, when virtue was equated with weakness, sweetness, innocence and sentimentality. Lack of education, of employment opportunities and of legal rights combined to help the woman accept the inevitability of her dependence on the man, and therefore the naturalness of the 'double standard'. In George Drysdale's words:

> If we examine the origin and meaning of these singular ideas with regard to women, we shall find that they are based upon no natural distinction between the sexes, but upon the erroneous views of man, and especially upon the mistaken ideas as to the virtue of female *chastity*. It is to guard this supposed virtue, that all the restrictions on female liberty and female development in body and mind have arisen.[31]

During the seventeenth and eighteenth centuries arguments were advanced to support the existence of the 'double standard' – principally that sexual freedom for women would introduce doubts about paternity and disturb inheritance laws and property rights. Such an argument was still being used in the mid-nineteenth century, although there was increasing recourse to the woman's innately sexless nature. W.R. Greg described the typical feelings of an ordinary woman on losing her virginity:

> What is, among the originally correct-minded and well-conducted, the real difference between the first sacrifice at the shrine of love in the case of a married and of an unmarried woman? It is not that the one feels that she is acting virtuously and the other that she is acting

> viciously – *the sense of shame is the same in both cases.* . . Among the decorously educated the first sacrifice is made and exacted, *in both cases,* in a delirium of mingled shame and love.[32]

The reference to education is significant, for a woman's purity although natural, had to be carefully guarded and sedulously nurtured. Ignorance was an essential component of innocence – 'the mere knowledge of the facts of sensuality often result in degradation of the mind'.[33]

Before the eighteenth century women had not been regarded as naturally sexless. An examination of popular books on marriage shows the way that the medical profession came to accept and propagate the new idea during the middle years of the nineteenth century. Ryan, in his discussion of marriage, decided that the female derived greater pleasure from the sexual act, even though the male had the more important role in reproduction, the semen actually imparting life to the ovum:

> In fine, the conformation of the sexes, enables the female always to receive, and never according to the expression of Solomon, to be satisfied and therefore sexual enjoyment is considered more delicious and protracted in one sex than the other. If we consider that the other sex have the nervous system much more sensitive than ours, the skin finer and more delicate, that their feelings are more acute, their mamae the seat of vivid sensibility from uterine sympathy, the nipples erected during intercourse, we must agree with Delignac that their enjoyment is more intense and extended through the whole economy, than in man, and that coition and impregnation generally excites in them a universal tumour in all parts of the body.[34]

Ryan followed a long line of medical writers, but his conclusions were based on up-to-date scientific reports. He considered that the woman was physically inferior, and agreed with contemporary opinion, that, because of menstruation and maternity, she was a natural invalid for most of her adult life:

> . . .women are more sensitive, weak, influenced by moral and physical causes, and more liable to diseases than the other sex. The constitution is more feeble, and is pecularly influenced by the mysterious process of reproduction, pregnancy, parturition, the puerperal state and lactation, as well as by the other function peculiar to it.[35]

William Acton's works evidence some of the changes in scientific knowledge that took place during the period 1840-65. He maintained, however, that a woman found little pleasure in the sexual act:

> I have taken pains to obtain and compare abundant evidence on this subject and the result of my inquiries I may briefly epitomise as follows: I should say that the majority of women are not very much troubled with sexual feeling of any kind. . . there can be no doubt that sexual feeling in the female is in the majority of cases in abeyance, and that it requires positive and considerable excitement to be roused at all; and even if roused (which in many cases it never can be) is very moderate compared with that of the male.[36]

According to Acton, woman existed to be man's helpmate and in the sexual field this meant being a suitable receptacle for 'the natural expulsion of semen', dutifully compliant but never exciting – as excitement might lead a man to commit health-damaging excesses. Women who did feel excitement were actually on the road to nymphomania – 'a form of insanity that those accustomed to visit lunatic asylums must be fully conversant with'. For this complaint Acton recommended excision of the clitoris.

Acton's views were not shared by all, and there were doctors who contended that sexual pleasure was natural in women. Dr Charles Routh, a leading gynaecologist, and others involved in the Isaac Baker Brown controversy over clitoridectomy in 1866, agreed that the clitoris was the seat of sexual pleasure in healthy women.[37] There seems, however, little doubt that Acton's views were widely accepted and well received by the profession at large. The entirely hostile reception accorded to a book which urged the equal strength of a woman's desires and the necessity for her socially approved expression illustrates how well Acton's book represented current opinion. Drysdale's *The Elements of Social Science,* first published in 1859, was a plea for total equality in society for women: he stressed the similarities rather than the differences between the sexes:

> In women exactly as in man, superior bodily strength, physical daring, and nervous power are indispensably requisite to form a fine character; and these are only to be obtained by strengthening the frame, and by training the nervous system to a healthy and elevated vigour. It is not true that the masculine and feminine virtues are frequently in contrast with each other. The two natures are built on

> the same original model and, in the main, they are alike in their laws.[38]

In order to enable a woman to enjoy her sex life without unwanted children, Drysdale advised the use of contraceptives. His book was coolly received by the *Lancet,* which considered that it advocated a licence for indiscriminate debauchery.

Woman's 'natural position' as man's helpmate and legitimate sexual outlet demanded that she did not threaten him by developing her own sexual desires, or in any way opposing his. In the Preface to the sixth edition (1875) of *The Functions and Disorders,* Acton remarked on the fearsome effect upon men and women's demands for independence:

> During the last few years, and since the rights of women have been so much insisted upon and practically carried out by the 'strongest minded of the sex', numerous husbands have complained to me of the hardships under which they suffer by being married to women who regard themselves as martyrs when called upon to fulfil the duties of wives. This spirit of insubordination has become intolerable. . . as the husbands assert. . . since it has been backed by the opinions of John Stuart Mill.[39]

Acton's insistence on the sexlessness of women suggests that he may have felt that there might be strong evidence to the contrary. Those, however, who encountered such evidence reacted by, if possible, denying it – indeed when Dr William Sanger questioned two hundred prostitutes in New York in 1858, he asked them why they had taken up prostitution. The majority gave 'inclination' as their reason. Horrified by this response, Sanger argued that they could not have meant what they seemed to be saying:

> . . . but it is imagined that the circumstances which induced the ruin of most of those who gave the answer will prove that, if a positive inclination to vice was the proximate cause of the fall, it was but the result of other controlling influences. In itself such an answer would imply an innate depravity, a want of true womanly feeling, which is actually incredible. The force of desire can neither be denied or disputed. . . But it must be repeated, and most decidedly, that without . . . some stimulating cause, the full force of sexual desire is seldom known to the virtuous woman.[40]

Later writers, like Dr Harry Campbell, did admit that there were divergent views among medical men on the subject of desire in women. After conducting his own survey, he concluded that 'the sexual instinct is much less in women than in man' and he was pleased to report that his findings were supported by Acton, Tain, Tilt and other gynaecological authorities.[41]

Although family limitation was coming to be practised by many middle-class couples,[42] there was little sympathy in the medical press for women who wished to have some control over their own fertility through the use of contraceptives, in spite of the suffering and danger which still attended normal childbirth. 'The womb of woman is an animal's', wrote Dr Augustus Gardner, in a diatribe against modern woman's shirking of her biological duty, 'which has an intense desire to conceive, and which is in a fury if it does not conceive'.[43] The use of contraceptive devices, he maintained, was far more dangerous to a woman's health than were repeated pregnancies. Many British and American doctors were influenced by the work of French medical men on the dangers of contraception,[44] particularly that of L.F.E. Bergeret, translated into English as *Conjugal Onanism* and frequently cited. Dr C.H.F. Routh, an outstanding gynaecologist who had studied with Semmelweis, addressed the Medical Society of London in 1878, and quoted Bergeret to prove that many cases of disease in men and women followed the use of the condom, cervical caps and douches.[45] Worse, perhaps, than the physical effects of such mechanical means of contraception was the morally debasing effect upon women of becoming 'the lewd plaything of our (masculine) vices'.[46] 'If men teach women vicious habits', continued Dr Routh, 'how can they be assured of their fidelity when assailed by a fascinating seducer? And may not even unmarried women taste of forbidden pleasures also, so that your future wife shall be defiled as you have known her.'

It was not only a woman's sexual behaviour which aroused the concern of doctors, but every activity she engaged in which might interfere with her primary biological purpose. Whatever a woman aspired to achieve, she could not be relieved from the basic task – the production and rearing of children. Furthermore, a woman who hoped to escape her destiny by competing with men in intellectual or artistic fields could never hope to achieve success, because of the periodic draining of her energy in menstruation and in pregnancy:

> . . . women are marked out by nature for very different offices in life from those of men, and . . . the healthy performance of her

special functions renders it improbable that she will succeed, and unwise for her to persevere, in running the same course at the same time with him. . . whether they come to be mothers or not, they cannot dispense with those physiological functions of their nature that have reference to that aim, however much they might wish it and they cannot disregard them in the labour of life without injury to their health.

thus Henry Maudsley pontificated in 1874.[47]

Adolescence was believed to be an especially dangerous period as any violation of the laws of the body at this period could lead inevitably to pain and disease in mature life, culminating in a traumatic and possibly fatal menopause.[48] As the major part of a woman's education took place during the period of the establishment of the menses, the excuse of the dangers of the onset of puberty was used to criticise attempts to improve a woman's education by claiming that any sustained physical or mental labour could weaken her for life. In North America Dr Edward Clarke, and in England Dr Henry Maudsley led the attack on the contemporary education of women.[49] They were answered respectively by Dr Mary Putnam Jacobi and Dr Elizabeth Garrett Anderson.[50] The latter very sensibly pointed out that physiological processes established themselves quite smoothly in healthy human beings. 'Are we', she enquired, 'to assume that all women are permanent invalids?' As to the argument that menstruation periodically handicapped them she wrote from her own observations:

When we are told that in the labour of life women cannot disregard their special physiological functions without danger to health, it is difficult to understand what is meant, considering that in adult life healthy women do as a rule disregard them almost completely. . . Among poor women, where all the available strength is spent upon manual labour, the daily work goes on without intermission, and as a rule, without ill-effects. For example, do domestic servants, either as young girls or in mature life, show by experience that a marked change must be made in the amount of work expected from them at these times unless their health is to be injured? It is well known that they do not.[51]

Lack of understanding of what menstruation actually was persisted into the early twentieth century,[52] and helped to make it easier for male physicians to regard women as peculiarly at the mercy of their physiological functions. In many ways women were regarded as being closer to children or idiots than adults, because of their lack of control over their emotions, and the predominance of feeling over reason in their minds.[53]

This examination of female sexuality has thus far concentrated on the male viewpoint – how did women themselves regard their own sexual nature? Did they accept the conventional view that they were sexually null? It has been recently argued that the views of Acton and his adherents were deliberately imposed upon the medical profession, whilst at the same time women continued to believe that they were passionate and sexually active.[54] Present evidence on this point is still scanty, though it is clear that some very well-known women, including Elizabeth Blackwell, protested against the views of Acton.[55] She herself believed that a woman's desires were even stronger than those of a man, and that sexual pleasure was even more essential to her happiness and overall well-being.[56] Sexual appetites and feelings, she asserted, were an inseparable part of total passion for both sexes, and could not be separated, quantified or satisfied in the simplistic manner recommended by many male members of the medical community.

Rejection of the male stereotypic view of female sexuality was becoming evident in a number of fields, particularly medical, where women attempted to assert themselves. The concluding section of this essay is devoted to a brief examination of such areas as medical education, nursing and midwifery, and the 'anti-medical' movement.

The demand for access to medical education by women,[57] beginning in the late 1850s, aroused the medical establishment to heights of greater anger and disgust than any other aspect of the campaign for changes in society's attitudes towards women. The *Lancet,* in particular, conducted a vitriolic campaign of 'unprecedented malignity'.[58] The case against women doctors rested firmly on two principal arguments: firstly that menstruation and pregnancy made women 'unfit to be entrusted with the life of a fellow creature',[59] and secondly that 'female purity would inevitably be destroyed in women learning anatomy and physiology, especially alongside male medical students'.[60] According to the male viewpoint, knowledge of the human body and its functions destroyed 'that fine gloss of innocence which not only added to women's charm but was an essential part of their real social role to preserve intact some of the finer ideals and illusions of the race'.[61] Any knowledge of the world could destroy female innocence but medical knowledge was thought to be even more devastating in its effects.[62]

A plea for women to enter medicine was published by Thomas

Markby in 1869. He considered that not all branches of medicine should be open to women, but only those which might be seen by the conventional man as suited to their powers and character, that is pharmacy, midwifery and paediatrics.[63] If his recommendations were to be accomplished, women would have to be admitted to the same medical schools as were men. This comparatively tempered and limited plea for women practitioners, nonetheless, was found by some to be quite unacceptable and out of the question. A knowledge of physiology was a basic necessity in all the recommended specialisms, and it was thought that no woman could ever fully comprehend physiology. Moreover, and more importantly, the admission of women students would be utterly unfair to the men who would be unable to achieve anything with the sight of women undertaking studies 'which only necessity renders other than barbarous and revolting'. According to an editorial in the *Medical Times and Gazette,* Markby's mind had been unfavourably influenced by the company of women.[64] Markby's assertion that female practitioners were needed because women wanted attendants of their own sex, especially in childbirth, was strongly criticised: '. . . it is mere womanish malice to cast any slur on women who seek men's aid in illness or childbirth. Women prefer the services of men because men are stronger, truer, more trustworthy, more merciful, less capricious and altogether more helpful than women to each other. . .'.[65]

There followed, nonetheless, a strong demand for women doctors and midwives from women who support a change in attitudes. Elizabeth Blackwell, for example, is said to have undertaken her medical course, not from intrinsic interest in medicine, but because she desired to serve humanity, and particularly her own sex.[66] Only a woman, it was felt, could understand her sex's complaints – and only a woman could treat members of her own sex without exploiting the dependent situation of the patient. Sexual exploitation, it was believed, was often a concomitant of the treatment of poor women by male doctors. Poor prostitutes were especially vulnerable to male pressure when forced to seek hospital treatment.[67] One of the most moving testimonies to the relief women felt in being able to seek aid from a female doctor was voiced by Josephine Butler, who consulted Elizabeth Garrett in 1869,[68] and who had refused, as had her mother, to have a male doctor assist at her confinements, because she did not want a man present. In a letter to a friend she revealed her innermost feelings:

> O, if men knew what women have to endure, and how every good woman has prayed for the coming of a change, a change in this. How

> would any modest *man* endure to put himself in the hands of a woman medically, as women have to do into the hands of men?. . . believe me, the best and purest feelings of women have been torn and harassed, and shamefully hounded for centuries, just to please a wicked *custom,* while those women who are not intrinsically noble and good are debased, insensibly, by such custom. . . this is what the tyranny of the medical profession has accomplished.[69]

As it became established that some female patients preferred to consult women doctors, the medical profession itself slowly began to recognise the contribution to be made by women. Elizabeth Blackwell believed that the crucial element in woman's nature was 'the spiritual power of maternity', a quality which was present in all women, even in those who had not borne children. The qualities of maternity were:

> . . . the subordination of self to the welfare of others; the recognition of the claim which helplessness and ignorance make upon the stronger and more intelligent; the joy of creation and bestowal of life; the pity and sympathy which tend to make every woman the born foe of cruelty and injustice; and hope, i.e. the realisation of the unseen, which fuses the adult and the infant, the future and the present.[70]

The narrow and superficial maternalism which prevailed among contemporary scientific men, in her opinion, made the presence of women among their ranks a necessity.[71]

Women were meanwhile attempting also to establish themselves in a number of paramedical roles. Although the nurse was, from the beginning, an assistant and subordinate to the doctor, there was considerable hostility among medical men towards the trained middle-class woman who was entering nursing in the decades following Florence Nightingale's success in organising nursing services in the Crimea. There were many reasons why medical men did not always welcome the new 'ladies' who came to work in the hospitals. Two important considerations were that many of the new nurses were of a higher social class than the doctors working in the same hospitals, and that doctors feared that such educated women would soon seek to undermine their authority.[72] Thus even those who accepted that the educated woman had a place in the hospital were determined to ensure that it was a closely confined, and precisely defined one. In a favourable review of Zepherina Veitch's *Handbook for Nurses for the Sick* (1870) the *British Medical Journal* remarked that 'one of the great dangers in affording ladies such an amount of professional knowledge as can only be gained in a hospital will be that they may be tempted to take too much on themselves and intrude upon the special province of the medical man'.[73] Nonetheless Miss Veitch gained the journal's commendation by her insistence that 'obedience was the hallmark of the good nurse'.[74]

Although the training of nurses had created concern among men, the prospect of trained and educated midwives aroused even greater hostility. The accepted way for a young doctor to build up a practice was to gain the confidence of the women in the family as an accoucheur, thereby establishing faith in his ability and encouraging members of the family to avail themselves of his services. During the 1860s the Ladies' Medical College was established under the auspices of the Female Medical Society to train well-educated women in midwifery and medicine. It was greeted with great enthusiasm by those wishing to extend employment opportunities for women, and by the male opponents of 'man-midwifery'.[75] Other medical men, however, opposed this development more because they saw such women as taking from them the lucrative upper and middle-class cases. They had, apparently, no objection to uneducated women being trained and licensed to work under medical supervision among the poor. Many medical men who strenuously opposed the possibility of women doctors were nonetheless favourable to the idea that trained working-class women would take off their hands the burden of unrewarding poor cases. When a Midwives' Act was finally passed in 1902, after much debate in the previous decade, midwives were placed under the control of medical men. They saw the midwife not only as an auxiliary but also as a woman whose role would soon disappear entirely as the demand for better medical care increased.[76] The Act made possible further professional aspirations, for it provided significant encouragement and, more importantly, a precedent for state registration of nurses.

A particular area in which women could show their resentment of medical attitudes towards their sex was to participate in popular anti-medical movements such as the campaigns to repeal the Contagious Diseases Acts,[77] the Anti-Vivisection League Movement,[78] and the anti-compulsory vaccination struggles.[79] The Contagious Diseases Acts aroused considerable opposition from women, because they were openly discriminatory in both their intention and operation. The high level of participation by women in the organisation and membership of these campaigns clearly indicates the general feeling that the medical profession was hostile to women's aspirations to social equality.

Thus during the latter part of the nineteenth century women campaigned, in the name of common humanity, against the 'double standard', by arguing against stereotypes of the compulsively sexual male and the naturally sexless female. Detailed explanation of the social processes involved in this movement fall outside the scope of this essay, which nonetheless has sought to map out what has been an area largely neglected by social historians. The essay has attempted to explain how beliefs regarding sexuality have been socially institutionalised, have served a social function, and preserved the *status quo* of male dominance. It is important to understand changes in beliefs regarding sexuality in the context of a relationship between the professionalisation process and the changing structure of sexual division in society. Since there became apparent a surplus of women over men, there thus followed pressures to open up new occupational opportunities for women. The new role of women may be seen as 'marginal',80 particularly as informal barriers were created to protect monopolistic claims of medical men. This essay thus underlines the need for further detailed studies to explore the ideologies of women – and particularly those of medical women – in relation to changes in social structure, medical and lay knowledge, and medical training.

Notes

1. For an examination of lay manuals which were used to provide women with knowledge of generation, sex and contraception see the essays by Janet Blackman and Angus McLaren in this volume. For a review of the literature regarding the ideas of the medical profession at this period see also Diana Scully and Pauline Bart, 'A funny thing happened on the way to the orifice: women in gynaecology textbooks', *American Journal of Sociology, 78,* 1972-3, 1045-50, reprinted in Joan Huber (ed.), *Changing Women in a Changing Society,* Chicago, 1973.
2. See Ann Douglas Wood, 'The fasionable diseases: women's complaints and their treatment in nineteenth century America', *Journal of Interdisciplinary History, 4,* 1973-4, 25-52; Jill Conway, 'Stereotypes of femininity in a theory of sexual evolution', *Victorian Studies, 14,* 1970-1, 47-62, reprinted in Martha Vicinus (ed.), *Suffer and Be Still: Women in the Victorian Age,* Bloomington, Indiana, 1972, pp. 140-54; Elaine and English Showalter, 'Victorian women and menstruation' *Victorian Studies, 14,* 1970-1, 83-9, reprinted in Vicinus, *op. cit.,* pp. 38-44; Carroll Smith-Rosenberg, and Charles Rosenberg, 'The female animal: medical and biological views of woman and her role in nineteenth century America', *Journal of American History, 60,* 1973, 332-56, and Charles Rosenberg, 'Sexuality, class and role in nineteenth century America', *American Quarterly, 25,* 1973, 131-54.
3. Keith Thomas, 'The double standard', *Journal of the History of Ideas, 20,*

1959, 195-216.
4. Jonathan Dymond, *Principles of Morality*, London, 1829, p. 351.
5. Barbara Bodichon, *A Brief Summary of the Most Important Laws Concerning Women*, London, 1854; and Erna Reiss, *Rights and Duties of Englishwomen – a Study in Law and Public Opinion*, Manchester, 1934.
6. Peter J. Cominos, 'Late-Victorian sexual responsibility and the social system', *International Review of Social History 8*, 1963, 18-48 and 216-50.
7. See particularly Roy M. Macleod, 'The Anatomy of State Medicine: Concept and Application', pp. 199-227, and Ruth G. Hodgkinson, 'Social Medicine and the Growth of Statistical Information', pp. 183-98, both in F.N.L. Poynter (ed.), *Medicine and Science in the 1860s*, London, 1968.
8. On this see M. Jeanne Peterson, *Kinship, Status and Social Mobility in the mid-Victorian Medical Profession*, PhD dissertation, University of California at Berkeley, 1972, pp. 331 and 346-7; and John C. Burnham, 'Medical specialists and movements towards social control in the progressive era: three examples', pp. 19-30, and 249-52, in Jerry Israel (ed.), *Building the Organisational Society – essays on associational activities in modern America*, New York, 1972. On the growing status of the medical profession, see the essay by Ian Inkster in this volume.
9. *Lancet*, 1862, *i*, 466. Note also Elizabeth Blackwell's comment: '. . . the progress and welfare of society is more intimately bound up with the prevailing tone and influence of the medical profession than with the status of any other class of men', in her *The Influence of Women in the Profession of Medicine*, London, 1889, p. 3.
10. *Medical Times and Gazette*, 15 August 1869, 176
11. B. Barker-Benfield, 'The spermatic economy: a nineteenth century view of sexuality', *Feminist Studies, 1*, 1973, 45-56.
12. William Acton, *The Functions and Disorders of the Reproductive Organs in Childhood, in Youth, in Adult Age and in Advanced Life, Considered in their Physiological, Social and Moral Relations*, 4th ed., London, 1865, p. 74.
13. Joseph F. Kett, 'Adolescent and youth in nineteenth century America', *Journal of Interdisciplinary History, 4*, 1973, 284. Alex Comfort in his *The Anxiety Makers*, London, 1967, lists and describes several of the more popular manuals.
14. Michael Ryan, *Prostitution in London, with a Comparative View of that of Paris and New York*, London, 1839, and H. Tristram Engelhardt, Jnr., 'The disease of masturbation: values and the concept of disease', *Bulletin of the History of Medicine, 48*, 1974, 234-48.
15. Acton, *op. cit.*, pp. 28-9.
16. 'Onanism' seems to have been the term used by medical writers to describe both homosexuality and masturbation. See V.L. Bullough and M. Voght, 'Homosexuality and its confusion with the "secret sin" in pre-Freudian America', *Journal of the History of Medicine and Allied Sciences, 28*, 1973, 143-55.
17. Francis W. Newman, *The Theory and Results of the Contagious Diseases Acts of 1864, 1866, 1869*, Bristol, 1870?, p. 6. See also Ryan, *op. cit.*, p. 84.
18. For a detailed analysis of this pamphlet see Robert H. Macdonald, 'The frightful consequences of onanism: notes on the history of a delusion', *Journal of the History of Ideas, 28* 1967, 423-31. See also Engelhardt, *op. cit.*, 235;

19. F. Lallemand, *On Involuntary Seminal Discharges*, translated from the French by William Wood, Philadelphia, 1839, p. 1.
20. Acton, *op. cit.*, p. 6.
21. *Ibid.*
22. *Ibid.*, p. 14.
23. *Ibid.*, p. 21.
24. *British and Foreign Medico-Chirurgical Review*, July 1857.
25. John Laws Milton, *Practical Remarks on the Treatment of Spermatorrhoea and Some Forms of Impotence*, London, 1855.
26. (George Drysdale), *The Elements of Social Science, or Physical, Sexual and Natural Religion*, 7th edn., London, 1867, p. 87.
27. *Ibid.*, p. 88;
28. See Macdonald, *op. cit.*, 429, and E.H. Hare, 'Masturbatory insanity: the history of an idea', *Journal of Mental Science, 108*, 1962, 1-25.
29. The *Lancet* for 1866 has accounts of the events leading to the closure of this clinic.
30. Carroll Smith-Rosenberg, 'Puberty to menopause: the cycle of femininity in nineteenth-century America', *Feminist Studies, 1*, 1973, 59.
31. Drysdale, *op. cit.*, p. 167. See also R.S. Neale 'Middle-class morality and the systematic colonisers', and his *Class and Ideology in the Nineteenth Century*, London, 1972, pp. 121-42. He describes a 'minority ideology' among the middle class of which Drysdale was a part.
32. W.R. Greg, 'Prostitution', *Westminster Review, 53*, 1850, 473.
33. *British Medical Journal*, 1870, *i*, 112. Peter J. Cominos discusses the contradictions inherent in the belief that women are naturally sexually innocent – see his 'Innocent Femina Sensualis in unconscious conflict in Vicinus (ed.), *op. cit.*, pp. 155-72.
34. Ryan, *The Philosophy of Marriage*, London 1837, pp. 152-3.
35. *Ibid.*, p. 112.
36. Acton, *op. cit.*, p. 112.
37. *Lancet*, 1866, *ii*, 495.
38. George Drysdale, *The Elements of Social Science, or Physical, Sexual and Natural Religion*, 11th edn., London, 1873, p. 172.
39. Acton, *op. cit.*, (1875 edn.), p. 142.
40. William Sanger, *A History of Prostitution . . .*, New York, 1859, pp. 488-9.
41. Harry Campbell, *Differences in the Nervous Organisation of Man and Woman: Physiological and Pathological*, London, 1891.
42. J.A. Banks, *Prosperity and Parenthood; a Study of Family Planning among the Victorian Middle-Classes* London, 1954.
43. Augustus K. Gardner, *Conjugal Sins against the Laws of Life and Health, and their Effects upon the Father, Mother, and Child*, New York, 1870 and 1875, p. 53.
44. On this see Angus McLaren, 'Some secular attitudes towards sexual behaviour in France, 1760-1860', *French Historical Studies, 8*, 1974, 604-25, his 'Doctor in the House: medicine and private morality in France, 1800-1850', *Feminist Studies, 2*, 1975, 39-54, and his 'Sex and socialism: the opposition of the French left in the nineteenth century', *Journal of the History of Ideas, 37*, 1976, forthcoming.
45. C.H.F. Routh, *The Moral and Physical Evils likely to follow if practices intended to act as checks to population be not strongly discouraged and condemned*, London, 1879 (reprinted from the *Medical Press and Circular*, October 1878). Routh also refers to the use of 'intra-uterine stems', devised originally to correct uterine displacement but 'also used by some ladies of high position, and continually worn by them, with a view to

prevent conception' (p. 9).

46. To those women who had medical reasons for not wishing to become pregnant too frequently, Dr Routh advised prolonged breast feeding and the rhythm method. Unfortunately, like many of his contemporaries, he did not understand the physiology of the menstrual cycle (it was not fully established until the 1930s), and he advised women wishing to avoid conception to have intercourse after the twelfth day of their cycle, or around the time of ovulation for most women.
47. Henry Maudsley, 'Sex in mind and education', *Fortnightly Review, 15* (new series), 1874, 466-83. For the effect of menstruation upon a woman's creative powers see Showalter and Showalter, *op. cit.*
48. Smith-Rosenberg, *op. cit.*, and Edward John Tilt, *The Change of Life in Health and Disease,* 2nd Edn., London, 1857.
49. Edward H. Clarke, *Sex in Education: or, a Fair Chance for Girls,* Boston, 1874, and Maudsley, *op. cit.*
50. R. Putnam (ed.), *Life and Letters of M.P. Jacobi,* New York and London, 1925, and Elizabeth Garrett Anderson, 'Sex in mind and in education: a reply', *Fortnightly Review, 15* (new series), 1874, 582-94. For an interesting discussion of the arguments of all four protagonists see *Westminster Review, 46* (new series), 1874, 456-99.
51. Anderson, *op. cit.*, 585.
52. See for example *Lancet,* 1878, *i,* 346-7. Adam Raciborski had established the connection between ovulation and menstruation in 1845. Vern Bullough and Martha Voght, in their 'Women, menstruation and nineteenth-century medicine', *Bulletin of the History of Medicine, 47,* 1973, 66-82, remark on the continuing acceptance of theories of menstrual cycle shown to be untrue.
53. *Lancet,* 1871, *ii,* 161-2.
54. Carl Degler, 'What ought to be and what was, women's sexuality in the nineteenth century', *American Historical Review, 79,* 1974, 1467-98.
55. See Linda Gordon's essay, 'Voluntary motherhood', in M. Hartmann and L.W. Banner (eds.), *Clio's Consciousness Raised: New Perspectives on the History of Women,* London, 1975, pp. 54-71.
56. Elizabeth Blackwell, *The Human Element in Sex. . . ,* London, 1882, p. 17.
57. On this see E.H.C. Moberley Bell, *Storming the Citadel. The Rise of the Woman Doctor,* London, 1953, and E. Lutzker, *Women Gain a Place in Medicine,* New York, 1969. On Elizabeth Blackwell see Rachel Baker, *The First Woman Doctor. The Story of Elizabeth Blackwell, M.D.,* London, 1946; P. Chambers, *A Doctor Alone: A Biography of Elizabeth Blackwell: The First Woman Doctor, 1821-1910,* London, 1956; and E.P. Link, 'Elizabeth Blackwell, citizen and humanitarian', *Woman Physician, 26,* 1971, 451-8. On Elizabeth Garrett Anderson see J.G. Manton, *Elizabeth Garrett Anderson: a woman among Victorians,* London, 1958, and L.G. Anderson, *Elizabeth Garrett Anderson,* London, 1959. On both these see N. St. J. Fancourt, *They Dared to be Doctors. Elizabeth Blackwell and Elizabeth Garrett Anderson,* London, 1965, and Nathan Roth, 'The personalities of two pioneer medical women. Elizabeth Blackwell and Elizabeth Garrett Anderson', *Bulletin of the New York Academy of Medicine, 47,* 1971, 67-79,
58. *Spectator,* 13 December 1870.
59. *Lancet,* 1858, *i,* 44.
60. *Lancet,* 1878, *i,* 18. This editorial describes medical education for women as 'violating the laws of decency'.
61. *Saturday Review, 20,* 1865, 602. See also the chapter on 'Love' in Walter

E. Houghton, *The Victorian Frame of Mind, 1830-1870,* New Haven, 1957, for a fuller exposition of this idea. For the medical case see J.N. Burnstyn, 'Education and sex: the medical case against higher education for women in England, 1870-1900', *Proceedings of the American Philosophical Society, 117,* 1973 (April), 79-89.

62. An interesting comment on the corrupting effects of knowledge is provided in the diary kept by A.J. Mumby, a barrister who befriended many working women. In the 1850s, when still a young man, he went to call on Louisa Baker, a twenty-two-year-old milliner. He commented, 'Louisa herself, though a virtuous respectable girl, has not – nor can any such girl have – that *ignorance of vice* which one desires in a lady'. See Derek Hudson, *Mumby. Man of Two Worlds – The Life and Diaries of Arthur J. Mumby 1828-1910,* London, 1972, p. 19.
63. Thomas Markby, *Medical Women,* London, 1869.
64. *Medical Times and Gazette,* 1874, *ii,* 191-2.
65. *Ibid.*
66. Bell, *op. cit.,* p. 30. See also the chapter by Sophia Jex-Blake in Josephine Butler (ed.), *Woman's Work and Woman's Culture,* London, 1869. Elizabeth Blackwell, an Englishwoman, gratuated in medicine in 1849 at Geneva Medical College, New York State, and ran a dispensary for women and children in the slums of New York. She returned to Britain to practise medicine, and was permitted to register under the Act of 1858, by virtue of having practised medicine before the qualifying date, 1 October of that year. As the only woman able to register, she was to be a leading campaigner for medical education for women. For further information on her life, see the sources cited in note 57 above.
67. Josephine Butler, *An Appeal to the People of England,* London, 1870, p.20. For an account of hospital treatment of women found to be in need of treatment under the Contagious Diseases Acts, see D. and J. Walkowitz, 'We are not beasts of the field: prostitution and the poor in Plymouth and Southampton under the Contagious Diseases Acts, *Feminist Studies, 1,* 1973, 73-106. See also E.M. Sigsworth and T.J. Wyke, 'A study of Victorian prostitution and venereal disease', in Vicinus, *op. cit.,* pp. 77-99, and for a general description of treatment practices see T.J. Wyke, 'Hospital facilities for, and diagnosis and treatment of venereal diseases in England 1800-1870', *British Journal of Venereal Diseases, 49,* 1973, 78-85.
68. Elizabeth Garrett was able to sit the examinations of the Society of Apothecaries, and in 1865 gained the L.S.A., as the 1815 Act only spoke of 'persons'. The rules were subsequently changed. She had served her apprenticeship at the Middlesex Hospitals – starting her studies as a nurse. After attempting unsuccessfully to study at St Andrews, she received her MD from Paris in 1870. The Marylebone Dispensary for Women and Children, which she founded, served the poor, while she practised also among the rich, and ultimately founded the New Hospital for Women solely for, and staffed by women. See Manton, *op. cit.*
69. Josephine Butler to 'Dear Friend', 22 February 1868, Josephine Butler Collection, Fawcett Library.
70. Blackwell (1889), *op. cit.,* p. 8.
71. Elizabeth Blackwell, *Erroneous Methods in Medical Education,* London, 1891, p. 7.
72. Brian Abel-Smith, *A History of the Nursing Profession,* London, 1960, p. 27. On Miss Nightingale's views, see Edward T. Cook, *The Life of Florence Nightingale,* vol. I, London, 1913 (especially chaps. III and IV), and Cecil Woodham-Smith, *Florence Nightingale, 1820-1910,* London, 1950.

73. *British Medical Journal*, 1870, *i*, 132. Miss Veitch was Head Surgical Sister at King's College Hospital. After her marriage she helped to establish the Midwives' Institute.
74. For an examination of the conflicts within the nursing profession, see Abel-Smith, *op. cit.*, particularly chaps. five and six.
75. Some men opposed male attendance at birth as an offence against female modesty. Those who opposed the use of the speculum for gynaecological examinations seem to have been motivated by the same feelings. The medical examination of women was referred to as 'instrumental violation'. Women's objections were qualitatively different in that they stemmed from a feeling very similar to the contemporary one, that speculum examination was a breach of the woman's sovereignty of her person – see Josephine Butler (1870), *op. cit.*, pp. 18-19. Dr James Edmunds, one of the founders of the Ladies' Medical College, argued that the training of female midwives would spare the modesty of women and, perhaps more significantly allow the doctor to spend more time in lucrative practice.
76. For a comprehensive and illuminating study in this neglected area see Jean E. Donnison, *The Development of the Profession of Midwife in England, 1750-1902*, PhD thesis, University of London, 1974. See also her forthcoming *Midwives and Medical Men*, London, 1977.
77. F.B. Smith, 'Ethics and disease in the later nineteenth century: the Contagious Diseases Acts', *Historical Studies, 15*, 1971, 118-35, and D. and J. Walkowitz, *op. cit.*
78. Richard D. French, *Anti-Vivisection and Medical Science in Victorian Society*, Princeton, New Jersey, 1975.
79. See for example Roy M. Macleod, 'Medico-legal issues in Victorian medical care', *Medical History, 10*, 1966, 44-9, his 'Law, medicine and public opinion: the resistance to compulsory health legislation, 1870-1907', *Public Law*, 1967, 107-28, and 189-211, and Royston J. Lambert 'A Victorian National Health Service: State Vaccination 1855-1871', *Historical Journal, 5*, 1962, 1-18.
80. On the concept of marginality see E.V. Stonequist, *The Marginal Man*, New York, 1927, and the essay by Ian Inkster in this volume.

5 MARGINAL MEN: ASPECTS OF THE SOCIAL ROLE OF THE MEDICAL COMMUNITY IN SHEFFIELD 1790-1850

Ian Inkster

The individuals who serve here as the basis for the collection and correlation of material were all concerned with advancing medical services or knowledge in a provincial and industrial setting which was undergoing vast changes throughout a period which has so often been termed revolutionary. Both victims and creators of circumstances, their individual social images and collective occupational interests served to determine many of their actions and beliefs, and it was the vigour with which the latter were projected which established their importance as a group in the development of Sheffield in this period. The intention of this paper is to describe and explain this social behaviour. The term 'medical' serves as the main parameter within which the historical material is analysed, but a principal theme of that analysis is the concept of social marginality. The man of medicine who had no established social status *vis-a-vis* his client was in an awkward siguation. For this reason alone, individuals who proclaimed medicine as their occupation were likely to be concerned with the complex and changing problem of their own social identity.

Of course, most of the 'new men' in the provinces were marginal to established English society if only because they were demonstrably mobile. They were on the move in terms of location, income and occupation. Their first reaction to their perceived siguation was to further remove themselves from such an established norm (itself as much perceived as real) by adopting a politics, a religion and a way of life which at once enhanced and gave power to their distinctiveness. As Thackray has recently shown, it might well have been such a profound social need which resulted in the growth of a provincial scientific culture in early nineteenth-century England.[1] But the medical men were marginal twice over, for they were both provincials striving for individual status, and members of a profession yet in the making.

The concept of the 'marginal man' was first suggested by Robert E. Park (1864-1944), a leader of what was to become known as the 'Chicago School' of sociologists. Park initially used the term in a paper on 'Human Migration and the Marginal Man', published in the *American Journal of Sociology* in 1927. The marginal man, for Park, was he who moves in more than one social world and is not completely at home in any.[2] Unfortunately, the early linking of marginality and culturally isolated migrant groups, created a tendency to unnecessarily limit the application of the term. Thus E.V. Stonequist, in his book entitled *The Marginal Man,* wrote only of racial marginality even though he recognised in passing that such groups as the *declasse,* the migrant from country to city, and women in a new role might fit the definition.[3] If the individual's conception of himself is not an individual but a social product, and if the process whereby self conception matures involves real social action, then the historian, faced with the problem of analysing a complexity of empirical data, might make use of the notion of social marginality in a fundamental manner. The material which follows suggests that marginality might explain the activities of specific groups within a national society quite as much as it does the actions of migrant groups moving across the frontiers of a national cultural and social system.[4]

Section I of the paper is concerned with professionalisation, which has been visualised as a minor concept feeding into that of marginality. Even in the London setting, the medical man was occupationally marginal, and it is argued below that one of the root causes of ambivalence was the working of the educational and training 'system'. The next section of the paper focuses upon the more fundamental marginality of *provincial* men, of which the medics were a small, extreme group, in that they were also within the category of non-industrial occupations which Sheffield harboured, and in many cases newly arrived. In addition they were a decidedly socially mobile group of men. Whilst it was the occupational interests of the medical men which forced the direction of their actions, the most important motivation for such actions – the need to establish a definite, identifiable social image – was never in doubt. Section III centres on the resulting alliance between the medical community and the industrial classes, an alliance which had a remarkable impact on the institutional and cultural history of Sheffield in the period before 1850. In this section, the activities of the group in voluntary associations serve not only as a measure of their influence but also of their need as a marginal group – that which Stacey has termed 'social comfort'.

In all this, the process of professionalisation is of utmost importance, for within the provincial context it was closely involved with the effort by medical men to legitimise their social and intellectual positions through social action. A fully professional group may have felt itself above reproach; a professionalising group was wholly aware of its sensitive social position.

I

The ideologies and activities of the provincial medical men can thus be partially interpreted in terms of the significant changes occurring in the areas of medical knowledge, training, qualifications and institutions on the national level. How far could the varied occupations grouped under the heading of 'medical' be termed professional? what sort of an image did medicine project within the larger society? and how did the provincial situation relate to that in London? It would appear to be fairly widely accepted that certain minimum criteria must be fulfilled in the process of professionalisation. These would include full-time practice, the high degree of skill or expertise of the member, explicit and fairly uniform educational and training programmes, recognised and consistent examinations leading to readily identified qualifications, legal recognition and autonomy of regulation in the areas outlined above. In addition, a certain number of less tangible criteria prove themselves as the process evolves: the development of a group consciousness finding expression in accepted organisations, a degree of self-control regulated by an ethical code, an orientation outwards as to the image or status of the member in the wider social context, and, to some extent following from all these, a recognition of the similarity of social class composition within the profession.

Greenwood has shown how these criteria may be categorised in terms of the *attributes* of an ideal profession and provides us with a measure as to the extent of professionalisation in medicine in the period prior to 1850.[5] The first attribute is that of systematic theory, the command of a fund of knowledge which in turn demands the existence of many of the criteria already mentioned, such as accepted educational and diffusion mechanisms and the development of critical attitudes. We will return to this attribute at a later point as it appears to be the basic one from which all others follow. The remaining four attributes of authority, the sanction of the community, the establishment of a code of ethics and the existence of a professional culture were undoubtedly yet to come to maturity at this time. At the beginning of the period, authority within the medical fraternity was ostensibly possessed by the three main corporations, the College of Physicians, the Company of Surgeons (from 1800 the Royal College of Surgeons), and the Society of Apothecaries. But without a system of registration such authority was nominal and not representative of control over the majority of practitioners. It is true that if an Edinburgh doctor of medicine wanted to practise in London he would first have to become a licentiate of the Royal College of Physicians, but on the other hand graduates of Oxford and Cambridge were completely exempt from membership of any body, and this was the case also with those who practised outside the metropolis.[6] Until the Act of 1815, the position of druggists and apothecaries was even more confused despite the fact that they represented roughly three-quarters of the total of medical men.[7] Whilst their positions of status and training were quite separate from the surgeons and physicians, the latter group were also in a state of flux, and this is perhaps best exemplified by the battle between the licentiates and the fellows of the College of Physicians. This established the point that hierarchical status and achieved status (through qualifications, medical discoveries and publications, etc.), were by no means aligned, and although the resulting pamphlet debate reached a height in the 1790s the issues were not really faced until the parliamentary committee of 1834.[8] If within a sub-group existing authority and status patterns were being challenged, this is even more true of the ralationship between the sub-groups. As late as the 1830s an MRCS had to undergo disenfranchisement if he was to become qualified for the LRCP. The cause of all this doubt and confusion was basic and one which lies at the heart of the concept of 'profession'; whilst sub-groups were legally defined into three layers with nine bodies combining (more or less) to solidify these into a definite hierarchy, the actual *practice* of the physician, surgeon and apothecary often greatly overlapped, and in some cases coincided.[9] The result, especially in the provinces, was the emergence of the general practitioner, whose more varied functions placed him in a quite different social position to his predecessor as he was increasingly likely to secure a wider social composition in the make-up of his patients, to be less reliant on the precarious demands of an influential few.[10]

Because of significant changes in the areas of organisation and the structure of authority, the medical practitioner did not on the whole gain the sanction of the community simply because the layman could not immediately identify the status of any one medical man. Of over one thousand medical men in London alone in 1817, only 92 were licentiates and 45 fellows of the College of Physicians, the rest being members of the apothecaries' and surgeons' bodies.[11] From 1834 the British Medical Association was advocating registration of all medical men together with preliminary examinations and uniform licensing. However, this early movement failed and as late as 1858 there existed nineteen separate licensing bodies in England. In this situation, the possibilities of the emergence of a common code of ethics and professional culture were not high. The sharing of values, norms, symbols, and the internalisation of these was made immensely difficult, especially when we consider the inclusion of at least three distinct social classes within the group promoting medicine. If we confine ourselves to occupational and income criteria alone (as distinct from status positions or conflict reaction to authority structures), then in many cases the apothecary and the medical instrument maker could be included in the labour aristocracy as 'artisans', the opticians, druggists (less fully trained than the apothecaries but, as wholesalers and retailers, often earning more income), dentists and most surgeons as within the 'middling classes', and the physicians, with some surgeons, as a service sector of the middle class. As we shall see, this social mix led to problems of identity in the provincial, urban setting.

Behind all this lay the changing pattern of medical education, for as Poynter has emphasised, 'medical education reflects the organisation of the profession and its institutions', and is an essential element in Greenwood's attribute regarding systematic theory.[12] It may be true that from the later 1830s, as Holloway claims, 'medical knowledge became more scientific, medical education more systematic, and the medical profession more unified'.[13] But even this is at best a partial truth for until the 1850s the Licentiate of the Society of Apothecaries, the Membership of the College of Surgeons and the Licentiate of the College of Physicians could all be obtained as the result of extremely varied systems and levels of training, involving universities, hospitals, dispensaries, provincial schools, private schools, societies and institutions, and systematic courses by independent public lecturers.

Up to the early nineteenth century the lack of a uniform system of medical knowledge meant that simplistic systems of a 'final cause' nature vied with each other in the educational field, e.g. humoral pathology. The sterility of this had two principal effects. The first was that by the 1790s the non-speculative empiricism of France had come to dominate the field, especially so, perhaps, in anatomy. The second was that, in an attempt to broaden medical education, certain teachers endeavoured to graft on formal instruction in closely related fields the most important of which, as we shall see below, was natural and experimental science. This was, then, an early attempt to establish a command over knowledge through breadth rather than through a universally accepted depth, and it was particularly the alliance thus forged between medical and scientific training that was so significant in the late eighteenth and throughout the subsequent century.[14]

Much further research is necessary before the extent of the variety of content and standards in medical education can be firmly established, yet, as has been argued, this is a vital area of historical interest if we are to measure the extent of professionalisation in medicine and the subsequent marginality of the medical community as a whole. If we consider developments centred around a small group of influential men in London, some idea of the complexity of the situation may be gained. A small group of innovators could with ease destroy uniformity. It was precisely these London teachers who provided the basic contact between metropolitan developments and the provinces; many provincial practitioners received the bulk of their teaching at the apprenticeship stage by attending courses of medical and scientific lectures, and many of these were given outside the 'normal' channels of the large hospitals.

The early eighteenth century saw the development of an extensive system of private lecturing in medical and allied subjects in London, and this was to continue in some strength to the end of our period. Caesar Hawkins (1711-86, FRCS), surgeon to St George's Hospital delivered courses of lectures on anatomy privately at Pall Mall Court in the 1730s at the same time as George Thompson was giving the same at the New Exchange in the Strand. Such courses were given in the mornings and evenings, and tickets were obtainable at the various coffee and chocolate houses.[15] A frequent lecturer in the same decade was Francis Nicholls MD who gave evening courses on both anatomy and physiology at his house in Lincoln's Inn Fields each day, and less frequently at Clare Market where syllabi were available.[16] Generally, courses cost between one and four guineas depending on the venue, length and lecturer. Similar public, independent lectures were given throughout this decade by William Broomfield (1712-92, surgeon to the Lock Hospital and St George's), Thomas Griffiths (surgeon of Cheapside), who included specific courses on neurology, Sir Richard Mannington (MD, FRS, on midwifery), William Hewitt and Nathan Alcock (1707-79, FRS).[17] Perhaps of most importance were those of William Lewis, (1708-81, MB, FRS), who lectured throughout the 1730s and 1740s at his Elabatory in New Street near Fetter Lane. As one of the foremost chemists of the age his medical and scientific lectures would have been most authoritative and particularly influential in the training of his students as they covered a wide field, including chemistry and pharmaceutical chemistry, and were delivered 'with a view to the Improvement of Pharmacy, Trades and the Art Itself'.[18] It was within this tradition that the medical lecturers of the later eighteenth century fell.

By the 1790s some of the most famous medical men of the day were involved in public lecturing, and, apart from those now well known, included William Turnbull (1729-96), George Pearson (1751-1828, MD,

FRS), William Blair (1766-1822, MRCS and surgeon to the Lock Hospital), Robert Hooper (1773-1835, MD, LRCP), George Fordyce (1736-1802, MD,FRS), Thomas Alcock and John Abernethy (1764-1831, FRS).[19] Courses were now much more ambitious. At his private laboratory in Whitcomb Street, George Pearson lectured on a variety of medical and chemical subjects and thus taught chemistry to W.T. Brande who himself became a chemical lecturer in London. Pearson later moved his laboratory to George Street where he continued lecturing on chemistry, natural philosophy and physic until well into the nineteenth century whilst holding his position as senior physician to St George's Hospital.[20] William Blair's courses covered anatomy, animal economy, anthropology and clinical practice and were given at his house in Great Russell Street, Bloomsbury, 'for the information of Scientific persons, Amateurs of Natural History, students in the liberal Arts, and Professional Men in general'.[21] The surgeon Charles Brown's lectures on anatomy and physiology were of a more popular nature. Delivered at the Westminster Assembly Rooms, they were possibly linked with the London Society for the Encouragement of Genius, of which he was president.[22] Perhaps the best example of public lectures of a popular type which yet strived to link systematic medical knowledge with science were those of Mr Hardie, a surgeon of Great Portland Street. He lectured at the Lyceum, at Somerset Street and at his own Experimental Philosophic Lecture Room and Theatre of Rational Amusement in Oxford Street, offering courses throughout the 1800s on experimental philosophy, astronomy, mathematics and galvanism.[23] Quite obviously then the variety of standards in the field of public medical and related lectures of an independent nature was very considerable, ranging from popular science bordering on quackery to ambitious medical courses by established teachers.

The popularity of the independent public lecture resulted in the formation of institutions designed to teach medical and related subjects, including full anatomical facilities. Up to the late 1820s the most important baker's dozen of these in the London area were as follows; the London Institution, the Medical Theatre in Burlington Gardens, the London Polytechnic, the Chemical Theatre at Windmill Street, the London Theatre of Anatomy and Medicine, the Western Literary Institution, the Anatomical Theatre at Blenheim Street, the Surrey Institution, the Anatomical School in Windmill Street, the Philomathic Institution, the Royal Institution, the Physiological Theatre in the Strand, and the Russel Institution, all of which offered their medical and scientific lecture courses to medical students,[24] and all of which were quite independent of hospital teaching or such hospital-affiliated medical societies as the Physical Society of Guy's Hospital.[25] A small group again dominated. George Pearson, who lectured independently on medical and chemical subjects, thus taught both Richard Phillips and William Thomas Brande. Phillips (1778-1851, FRS, FLS) then went on to give chemical lectures at the Lock Hospital, independent courses at his house at Cheapside, pharmaceutical courses at the London Theatre of Anatomy and Medicine, science lectures at the London Institute, as well as being prime founder of the science-orientated Askesian Society and a provincial itinerant science lecturer of renown.[26] Brande himself underwent medical training as an apprentice and as a pupil at both the Anatomical School and the Chemical Theatre in Windmill Street, then taught chemistry at the Medical Theatre in Burlington Gardens (founded and run by Robert Hooper, the medical lecturer), St George's Hospital and the Russell Institute, before taking up his position at the Royal Institution.[27] Members of the same group were also predominant in the diffusion of knowledge. George Fordyce, who had lectured on chemistry and medicine in the 1790s, was a founder of the Society for the Improvement of Medical and Chirurgical Knowledge, edited the *Medical Communications* (1784) and contributed many papers to the *Philosophical Transactions.* S.F. Simmons, who had lectured on anatomy in the 1780s and brought out his *Medical Register* in 1783, was another founder of the same society and the spirit behind the *London Medical Journal* of 1781. Richard Phillips was co-editor of the *Annals of Philosophy.*[28]

The multiple activities of such a small group illustrate that there existed a great variety of training and diffusion facilities outside of more established avenues, and that the potential provincial practitioner was subject to a host of diverse influences at a time in his life when he was most liable to be affected. This microcosmic approach also shows how the situation in London would have provided at best a marginal occupational identity for those who came within its influence, many of whom then moved on to establish themselves in an industrial provincial setting itself in the throes of an identity crisis.

II

The following account of medical men in Sheffield is limited to 120 individuals practising in the period 1790-1850, and includes surgeons, physicians, druggists, apothecaries, dentists, midwives and surgical instrument makers. This figure does not represent all those who lived by some medical skill in the town through this period, but only those who resided there for some time and who took some active part in the promotion of local medical activities. While they would number only a dozen or so in the 1790s, by 1825 the local directory listed 25 surgeons living in the town, and by 1837 this had risen to 44. In fact, most physicians and surgeons entered in the directories are included here, but this is true only of a small proportion of total practitioners in the other related field mentioned above. A glance at the local directories testifies to an accelerating growth in the numbers of medical men, this in direct response to the demands of the developing industrial region.

The reasons for such industrial development are not readily uncovered, although a traditional account in terms of local resources, market conditions and technological advances can be given, always bearing in mind that none occurred in any economic vacuum and that all were closely interrelated through time.[29] Local limestone, timber for charcoal and the streams of the Don, Sheaf and Porter providing power for wheels, hammers and mills, ensured that there was some growth of metal working industry in the region before the time of the first technical innovations. Up to the 1730s London merchants conducted most of the metal manufacture, and the later characteristic predominance of small shops and enterprises emerged at about this time, when Sheffield was producing and exporting one and a half thousand tons of goods to Doncaster and Hull annually.[30] The later years of the century witnessed a series of vital, localised innovations; the silver plating discoveries of the 1740s, the development of fusion plating for silver and Sheffield plate and the consequent rise of the die-cutter as the most skilled of artisans in the next decade, improvements in polishing hardened steel and in refining precious metals in the 1760s, the replacement of hammering by machine rolling of iron and steel at the turn of the decade, and the revolutionised process of working cast steel by reducing the bar to a fluid state in the 1770s. The diffusion of steam power for grinding completed this early series.[31] The canal developments of 1751-1815 eventually served to open up the Don, Trent and Humber as channels for Swedish, Russian and German ore, English and Scottish cast and wrought iron, and Newcastle steel, until the 1780s saw the real emergence of Sheffield forges for the manufacture of shear and other steels. Enclosure and immigration, together with natural population growth, served to adjust labour supply and augment the market potentialities of the region.[32]

Between 1736 and 1801 the population of the six townships increased by three and a half times, doubled between 1801 and 1831

(91,692), and trebled between 1801 and 1851 (135,300). This swift population growth, together with the industrial nature of the locality, meant that the professional and service group was very much in a minority, both in terms of the total population and of the industrial middle class. Yet it was the members within this group who were to play a large part in the total institutional development of the town. The position of the non-industrial occupations is illustrated roughly by a breakdown of census figures for 1831, based on a total population of 91,692, with the number of males over twenty-one years at 23,043. On a township basis the latter may be broken up into seven groups as follows; (a) males in manufacture, 10,955; (b) in trade and handicrafts, i.e. masters and journeymen, 6,452, (c) merchants and professionals, 1,234, (d) employees of (a + b + c), 2,640, (e) servants, 99, (f) labourers in agriculture, 418, and (g) other males, i.e. retired and unemployed, 1,013.[33]

Table 1. Numbers and Distribution of non-Industrial Occupations (1831)

Township	Total Males	(a + b + d) Total Males	c Total Males	c Total Population
Sheffield	15,455	89.4	4.9	1.3
Ecclesall	3,397	80.7	6.8	1.6
Brightside	1,860	84.0	6.1	1.3
Nether Hallam	1,107	81.8	6.1	1.4
Attercliffe	958	90.6	3.4	0.9
Upper Hallam	266	56.4	0.4	0.1
TOTAL:	23,043	87.0	5.35	1.3

Not only was the non-industrial professional and service group in a distinct minority, it was also distributed fairly evenly between the townships, suggesting that, even at this fairly late date, the authority and status of its members were by no means established. Throughout our period, the significant activities of this group could be made effective only through an alliance with the industrial middle class, and it is this which both explains and defines their social role, and in turn adds to an understanding of religious, political and cultural developments in the town.[34] Within the minority group lay the medical men.

Both marginality and mobility are illustrated by a brief examination of the backgrounds and careers of local medical men. Hall Overend, who became a leading local surgeon, was the son of a Sheffield clerk, served his apprenticeship with a local apothecary and represented much of the radical political interest in the area before 1830. His eldest son was educated at the grammar school, became FRCS and JP as well as gaining a reputation as one of the most accomplished surgeons in the provinces. Another son was articled to a solicitor, then attended Lincoln's Inn, 'finished' his education at Hamburg and was called to the Bar in 1837. He twice sought to become an MP for Sheffield in the Tory interest and was Chairman of the Royal Commission on Trade Outrages which sat at Sheffield in 1867. Joseph Law was the son of a local silversmith and was apprenticed to a local surgeon before his studies at London, Dublin and Edinburgh. He commenced his medical career in 1834 when he was appointed house surgeon to the Sheffield Dispensary, and in 1852 took his MD degree, thereafter practising in the town as a physician. William Marsden was the son of a local victualler and became first a pharmacist, then MRCS in 1827 and finally a doctor of medicine and well-known physician. Unlike the above men, Henry Jackson stemmed from an established line of local surgeons, he himself beginning to practise as such in the 1820s and securing an enviable reputation through his work at the Infirmary. His eldest son, born in 1839, was educated at the Sheffield Collegiate School, Cheltenham College and Trinity College, Cambridge, of which he was made fellow and tutor in 1864, becoming Regius Professor of Greek in 1906. Henry's youngest son, born 1843, was also educated at Cheltenham, then at Sheffield Medical School and the Infirmary, and finally at St Bartholomew's. He took over his father's practice in 1866 and extended it considerably. Such examples of upward mobility in and through medicine can be multiplied with ease: Charles Favell was the son of a man-midwife, became a surgeon in Sheffield and was an adamant Unitarian, but his son went to Cambridge and became deacon and later archdeacon of Sheffield; the surgeon John Sterndale was the son of an apothecary and the father of a poet; John Barber, the son of a pharmacist and the father of a very successful banker.[35]

In order to obtain both reward and status the medical man had to appeal to the community. This is well illustrated by the position of George Calvert Holland in 1832. Born in 1801 he was the son of a local artisan and spent his early years as a barber whilst teaching himself languages and the classics. In 1823 he left Sheffield for medical study at Edinburgh, spent most of 1825 in Paris attending medical and scientific courses, and graduated Bachelor of Letters of Paris in 1826, and MD of Edinburgh in 1827. During his four years in Scotland he was

President of both the Hunterian Medical Society and the Royal Physical Society. His first book, of 1829, was reviewed with favour in the *New Scots Magazine,* the *Edinburgh Literary Gazette* and in various medical journals, and by 1832 he was already nearing completion of his two volume *Enquiry into the Principles and Practice of Medicine.*[36] In addition to such obvious achievements in medicine he had from 1825 made serious efforts to establish himself in the purely local context, through his activities in the Literary and Philosophical Society, his support of both the Mechanics' Library and the proposed Mechanics' Institute, and by means of the important friendships made within the influential groups of Unitarians and political radicals.[37] By 1832 his Sheffield practice was worth £1,400 annually. Yet despite all this, his application for the position of physician to the Infirmary in April of that year was by no means a formality. In three columns of the local newspaper he presented his case, addressing himself to the governors and the 'ladies and gentlemen' of the town:

> I embrace the present opportunity of laying before you the following Testimonials; the opinions of different Medical Reviews and the Physiological Works I have published, and an account of the opportunities I have enjoyed for the acquisition of professional knowledge. The studies enumerated, are in addition to those I pursued in the University of Edinburgh, during a residence of four years – studies in nowise necessary to confer the privelege of Graduation. I am induced to present them in order to show, that I have long and zealously cultivated the profession to which I am warmly attached, and the various branches of Science and Literature with which it is intimately or remotely connected; I, therefore, hope I may be allowed to look forward to your liberal support on the day of Election, with no undue presumption.[38]

This was the critical moment for Holland's acceptance, and from thence his social future was assured. Thus, in 1833 he was made President of the newly formed Mechanics' Institute, two years later he was elected to the same office in the Literary and Philosophical Society, became town councillor and later alderman, which position he held until his death in 1865. Through his social actions, Holland established an image which coincided with, indeed epitomised, that held by the groups coming to power and influenced in the local context. As has been suggested, his successful career was mirrored by others.

The first sphere of activity in which medical men engaged was, obviously enough, the development of medical facilities and institutions, and the diffusion of medical knowledge, and this at once brought them into close contact with the industrial middle class. The initial major public enterprise in the medical field was the Sheffield Infirmary, opened in October 1794 with a local subscription of £17,500. Four years previously, William Young, a physician newly established in the town distributed three hundred copies of an anonymous circular signed 'A Friend of General Infirmaries' which strongly urged the importance of such an institution to local industrialists. In the next year a subscription was started, although the first regular meeting was that of 23 April 1792 when a committee was formed in order to extend the appeal in the belief that 'from the particular kind of Manufacture carried on in Sheffield and its Neighbourhood, an Infirmary near this Place would be extremely advantageous'. At that meeting 29 subscriptions worth £2,625 were obtained and two days later the committee could report a total figure of £6,937 obtained from 125 subscribers. A survey of the 33 persons donating £100 or more shows that a cross-section of the wealth of the town was involved.[39] Henceforth the Infirmary served as an institutional focus for the medical community, a physician or surgeon to the Infirmary was not simply the holder of a medical office, but also the approved representative of the local middle class and, as we have seen above, such approval was not easily granted.[40] Similarly, the Sheffield Jennerian Society, formed in March 1803, gained support far beyond that of the medical community and, in fact, its first 15 committee members did not include one medical man, being composed of three clergymen, one lawyer, one 'gentleman' whose future rested on the refining of sugar, two members of a long established family of ironmasters, and eight more newly settled local manufacturers.[41]

The encouragement of facilities for the securing and diffusion of medical knowledge required further local support. The tradition of the itinerant popular medical lecturer went back to the earlier eighteenth century, and Sheffield appears to have had its due quota. In 1761 the Chevalier Taylor was offering his 'Academical Oration on the Eye' to the local gentry, and in the next year R.B. Shapee distilled a form of knowledge alongside his medicines and cures. By the end of the century the local medical fraternity could demonstrate its contempt for such an approach. When J. Baylis arrived in the town in March 1791 to offer his lectures on animal electricity and his cures through the manipulation of the imperceptible fluid he was openly opposed: 'J. Baylis is sorry to hear that some of the Faculty have done everything in their Power to set this admirable science in the worst point of view, and that some gentlemen, who (with the vulgar) bear the appelation of Philosophers, are as inconsistent and averse to reason . . .'.[42] By the turn of the century the local men began to give their own public courses in an attempt to raise the status of medical knowledge to that of a fundamental science. In February 1807 Dr David Daniel Davis announced his intention of delivering a course of lectures 'upon several subjects connected with the health, habits and pursuits of this large and populous town'. His six lectures on the 'animal economy' were attended by audiences 'numerous and of the highest respectability', and composed of merchants and industrialists as well as medical men.[43] Medicine as a subject of study was also entering the local literary and scientific associations. For instance, the Society for the Promotion of Useful Knowledge, founded in January 1804, explored such topics as 'What is Instinct?', 'Whether is an uniform regularity of abstimiousness or an occasional deviation therefrom, most conducive to health', 'The Structure of the heart', 'A Case of Morbid Sensitivity' before dissenting ministers, lawyers, merchants and manufacturers.[44] The first lecture to the Society for Literary Conversation in 1806 was delivered by Davis under the title 'Connections between Anatomy and Physiology'.[45] The emergence of a general interest in medicine bore fruit in the formation of societies explicitly designed to provide such knowledge as well as to more formally train the intending practitioner.

The first society of this type to draw support from local manufacturers was the Humane Society, formed at the end of 1809 and led by most of the local medical men for the purpose of disseminating knowledge of such subjects as suspended animation and hydrophobia.[46] This was followed by the Sheffield Medical and Surgical Society established in 1820 and meeting regularly at the Angel Inn, at which medical men gave papers on problems especially relevant to the Sheffield trades, such as the grinders' asthma.[47] In 1828 two new medical societies were formed in competition with one another, both of them claiming to repesent the local medical community, and both attempting to secure adherents from the industrial middle class. On 14 February of that year the medical men of Sheffield, let by Drs Arnold Knight and Hall Overend, held a public meeting at the Cutler's Hall 'to consider the expediency of establishing an institution in connection with proper rooms for the delivery of professional lectures; to be accompanied with scientific demonstrations and experiments on the principles and properties of surgery and the Materia Medica'. Immediately, a group headed by Overend and Dr Corden Thompson began the conversion of the existing anatomy museum erected behind Overend's house in Church Street into what was henceforth called the Sheffield School of Anatomy and Medicine, which received its opening address from Thompson in October 1828. A second group headed by Knight and Dr Charles Favell elected to erect a new building in Surrey Street, and upon the raising of £2,000 by local subscription, this was opened as the Sheffield Medical Institution in July 1829. The identity forming function of such associations was adamantly proclaimed by both institutions. The intention of the Medical Institution was to promote

> . . .a greater unanimity of feeling amongst the members of the Profession. . .individual improvement by the mutual interchange of thought and the friendly discussion of Medical Subjects. . .and thirdly, the improvement of Medical Pupils by affording them facilities of acquiring knowledge which they did not before possess, by offering them opportunities of obtaining all their elementary education in the country.

In his address before the alternative society, Thompson stressed the ethical function of the educational process itself; how, for the individual pupil

> It will evince that he has something more to accomplish than the mere passing of an examination, or the obtaining of a licence to practice; that the possession of this, in fact, is but his passport to an entrance on a more extended and arduous course of labours; his title to the assumption of higher duties and responsibilities.[48]

Both societies were successful in capturing the attention of the public. The Church Street School appealed to a wide audience in its advertisements, and its chemistry lectures in particular were attended by both merchants and manufacturers, the most popular being those of Edward Barker, himself involved in several manufacturing enterprises. Lecturers to the Medical Institution included a lawyer, a professional chemist and the master of the local academy, and such subjects as moral philosophy, drawing and perspective, and veterinary surgery were a normal part of the total programme.[49] Up to 1850 there were at least four such separate medical societies (the Sheffield Medical and Chirurgical Book Society was established in 1834) engaged in producing medical facilities and knowledge and hence constantly bringing into contact medical and other interests.[50]

A result of all this was that certain important local coteries and informal associations came increasingly under the influence of medical men. Of the thirty-eight papers read before the Society for the Promotion of Useful Knowledge in the period January 1804 to November 1805 seven were on medical subjects, and medical men took a foremost part in non-medical, especially scientific, discussions. At the conclusion of a long lecture concerning controlled experiments on starch 'the theory was opposed as improbable, fanciful and founded upon no facts, by Messrs Overend and Moorehouse', both of whom are surgeons.[51] Although the Sheffield Book Society (founded in 1806) included such major merchant-manufacturers as Joseph and Samuel Bailey, John Marshall, Thomas Asline Ward, Edmund Wilson and William and Samuel Butler, it was completely dominated by medical men in terms of total membership, meeting places and books circulated.[52] The medical community was establishing a platform. These developments reached their height in the formation of the Physiological Society, which originated jointly with the merchant Thomas Ward and the physician George Holland, and held its first meeting in May 1837. Addressed to all 'literary and scientific gentlemen' its purpose, as declared in the first resolution, was to be 'the communication of knowledge on the important functions of life, by means of popular lecturers, reading of papers, and discussions monthly'. Apart from Holland as President, the first committee of eight was composed of one general wholesale merchant, one hosier who was also an ale dealer, one razor manufacturer, one Britannia Metal manufacturer, one hatter, one artist and drawing master, one knife and steel manufacturer and one tradesman.[53]

Through its overt occupational activities, the medical community had, by the 1830s, forged definite contacts and social relationships with a fairly wide cross-section of the society. Contemporaneously, the further stage in the establishment of a social image was more profound, extended well beyond occupational interests, and engendered a complex of social roles.

III

By the 1820s members of the medical community in Sheffield were turning towards an analysis of the local context of health problems. In the first year of the decade Dr Arnold Knight delivered a paper before members of the Medical and Surgical Society on the subject of the grinders' asthma which showed 'that out of 2,500 grinders, there are not 35 who have arrived at the age of 50 years, and perhaps not double that number who have reached the age of 45'. William White estimated that by the mid-1830s three-quarters of all grinders were engaged in steam wheels and that this served to vastly increase the incidence of asthma 'for he now works 10 or 12 hours a day on the average' when previously he had more choice and his work was halted 'in seasons of little water'.[54] As early as 1816 the merchant T.A. Ward had similarly pointed to steam and the work place as a deadly combination:

> We have had grinders between 60 and 70 years old, but they had the usual complaint of an asthmatic nature. Their particular branch, table knives, is salubrious, when compared with that of the fork-grinders, whose stones do not run in water, who grind dry, and are exposed to the flying particles of grit and steel, which reach their lungs and kill them at about 42 – you know John Fox – his son told me he knew only one instance of his men's reaching the age of 52. Some grinders fancy that hard drinking and fat meat may be serviceable by forcing down the noxious particules, but it is not the stomach which is injured but the lungs.[55]

The health hazard of dry grinding became the focus for a more general medical critique of local industrial working conditions and public provisions. In 1822 a public meeting was arranged by Arnold Knight and John Sterndale, both leading local medical men, in order to raise funds for J.H. Abraham and the financing of his invention of a magnetic filter for dry grinding waste, and such medical support was offered throughout the decade for subsequent inventions.[56] In 1833, Knight suggested in a paper before the Literary and Philosophical Society that criminals might be gainfully employed in dry grinding.[57] Five years later G.C. Holland made an important impact with his thorough paper to the same society under the title of 'Introductory Remarks to an Inquiry into the Social, Intellectual and Moral Condition of the Working Class' which surveyed working conditions in the cutlery trades and then went on to lampoon the Infirmary, Dispensary, National and Lancasterian Schools and the Society for the Better Condition of the Poor as local institutions for the welfare of the people. A few months later the physician published an extended version of this which concentrated on conditions of work.[58] At the same time he and Favell (see above) joined forces in an attack on the medical charities of the area, again addressing the Philosophical Society and thus many persons concerned with those charities. In 1841 Holland presented a long paper before the Statistical Department of the British Association for the Advancement of Science on the theme of 'The Vital Statistics of Sheffield' in which he acknowledged the help of 'a local committee' especially formed to prepare material. In the next year he persuaded the Literary and Philosophical Society to devote some of its funds to rewards for dry grinding inventions and published his highly critical and extremely detailed *Mortality of Grinders.* In 1843 his researches reached their critical peak with his lecture of January to the Philosophical Society on 'An Inquiry into the Condition of the Cutlery Manufacture in Sheffield' which was the final inducement to the town trustees in commissioning him to publish his large volume *The Vital Statistics of Sheffield.*[59]

The *Vital Statistics* is a fine example of the medical man as social critic; as a result of the book's findings Holland felt it necessary to resign his position at the Infirmary simultaneous with its publication. By this time, then, members of the medical community were taking up a definite and confident social stance.[60] It is hardly surprising that men in other spheres of life should associate with them and in turn be influenced by them. The point emphasised in this paper, and rehearsed repeatedly, is that such influences were made concrete through social actions. A table of the religious and political profiles of 20 leading[61] medical men suggests the social image being projected at the local level; it was through such political and religious affiliations that they came into even closer and more influential contact with the rest of the community.

Clearly, the most socially important of local medical men were also the most radical and distinctive in terms of religious and political affiliations.[62] Nor were they at all unrepresentative of the medical community (i.e. of the total 120 men) as a whole – rather, they epitomised it. For instance, as early as 1795, William Frith, Sheffield surgeon, a member of the Constitutional Society accused Henry Redhead Yorke, in a trial for conspiracy and treason, as being altogether 'too mild a man'.[63] By 1809 the medical fraternity represented a large part of the radical community, as illustrated in the support given G.C. Wardle, Francis Burdett and William Cobbett in their attempts to reform parliamentary procedure and expose corruption.[64] The preliminary meeting of the Sheffield Political Union, agitating for a general reform was dominated by such leading men as Holland, Knight and Evatt, but also very strongly backed by more humble and newly-arrived men like John Green, surgeon, and George Johnson, surgical instrument maker.[65]

The medical men had thus moved from a mainly implied radicalism through social medicine to a more explicit or formal radicalism through affiliation with identifiable (i.e. image producing) religious and political movements. Other individuals in Sheffield were adopting precisely the same attitudes, and the merging of these interests was a crucial process

Table 2. Profiles of the Medical Elite

Name	Occupation	Religion	Politics[66]
Barber, J.	Apothecary	Quaker	1790s Republican
Boultbee, H.	Surgeon	Unitarian	1830s Radical
Browne, J.	Physician		1780s Radical
Davis, D.	Physician	Unitarian	1810 Reformer
Deakin, R.	Surgeon	Congregationalist	
Earnest, R.	Physician	Unitarian	1810 Reformer
Ellis, T.	Med. Instr.	Quaker	
Evatt, W.	Dentist	Unitarian	1830s Radical
Favell, C.	Physician	Unitarian	1830s Radical
Favell, J.	Surgeon	Unitarian	1810 Reformer
Holland, G.C.	Physician	Unitarian	1830s-40s Radical
Jackson, H.	Surgeon		1810 Reformer
Knight, A.	Physician	Roman Catholic	1830s Radical
Moorehouse, J.	Surgeon	Rationalist	1810 Reformer
Overend, H.	Surgeon	Quaker	1810 Reformer
Staniforth, W.	Surgeon	Unitarian	
Sutcliffe, R.	Apothecary	Quaker	1790s Republican
Thompson, C.	Physician	Unitarian	1830s Radical
Warwick, T.	Physician	Unitarian	1790s Republican
Younge, W.	Physician	Unitarian	1780-1810 Reformer

in the social and cultural development of the town. When in 1826 the Friends of Civil and Religious Liberty met to honour Henry Brougham, discussants included the physician Arnold Knight and the surgeon John Sykes alongside Luke Palfreymen and Edward Barker, both of whom had already been seen to have been closely connected with the medical community. Other leading members of this small group included Samual Shore, ironmaster, merchant and banker, Joseph Read, silver refiner, Robert Gainsford and Charles Fenton, partners in silver and plating manufacture and Benjamin Sayle, ironmaster. Such examples of common political interests cutting across occupational and wealth boundaries can be found throughout the period, but especially in the 1820s and 1830s.[67]

The impact of the medical community was felt through the medium of voluntary associations in areas which not only included medicine, religion and politics, but also science, education, literature, charities and recreations, and it was this impact that was both wide and fundamental, especially when we consider the social characteristics of the whole medical community in Sheffield. The sociological significance of a study of voluntary associations is made clear by Margaret Stacey in her study of social life in Banbury:

> A study of voluntary associations shows chosen interests and chosen relationships: the type of interest for which people choose to associate and the social characteristics of those with whom they choose to associate. In other words, a man may choose to join a cricket club rather than a musical society because that is what he is interested in; and he may choose to join one cricket club rather than another because, he says, 'the members (of the second club) are not my sort' or because the club 'has not got a good atmosphere'. In short, he is looking, not only for an outlet for his interests, but also for the social comfort of mixing with those with whom he has most in common.[68]

If we substitute 'he can identify' for 'he has most in common' then the significance of the voluntary association in our historical context becomes fairly obvious. Marginal men felt the need to identify with a social image (or a series of social images) and they did so through committees, donations and public addresses. If we can agree with J.F.C. Harrison that by the later 1830s 'The middle classes of early Victorian Britain were aware of themselves to a greater degree than in the past', we can also emphasise that such awareness was a result of a long-term social process.[69]

Obviously enough, the medical community spanned many local voluntary associations and a complete representation of all memberships, even if possible, would be both lengthy and perhaps pointless. What is of most interest is the local influence of medical men. If, from the 120 in the group, we extract the 43 most important men in terms of both medical and social activities this serves to narrow the field.[70] Moreover, as simple membership does not necessarily presume 'influence', only the following three types of involvement have been considered; founders and first subscribers, those on committees for more than one year or holding meaningful posts requiring real duties, e.g. voluntary librarian, and those contributing to basic activities where the contribution required effort or preparation, e.g. the delivery of lectures and papers.[71] From a survey on this basis it was found that the 43 men ranged over 29 major voluntary associations through 193 distinct connections, i.e. on the average each association contained seven of the 43 men in influential positions. Of this group 22 were involved in the Literary and Philosophical Society, 18 in the Mechanics' Institute, and nine in the Friends of Parliamentary Reform. (A list of the institutions and extent of involvement is given in the appendix.) As before, the leaders appear to represent the general medical community: of 30 surgeons and physicians in Sheffield in 1825 exactly half were involved in the activities of the Literary and Philosophical Society in the year 1824-5; of 44 in 1833, 23 were active members of the newly formed Mechanics' Institute.[72]

One of the more unexpected of the associations dominated by the medical men was the Sheffield Mechanics' Institute, and its early history may serve to illustrate their persuasive influence. Over a number of years, the Institute emerged from a more modest project, the Sheffield Mechanics' Library, which included several medical men on its list of subscribers. At an annual meeting of the library in July 1831 both Luke Palfreyman and George Holland spoke on the possibility of conversion to a more ambitious format. Physicians Favell, Knight and Holland all gave lectures before members in an effort to raise funds and when Favell delivered his successful one on Humphrey Davy in November of that year

> The lecture was highly applauded by a numerous and attentive auditary; and it is to be hoped that the appeal made by the lecturer to the usefulness of Mechanics' Institutes will be the means of inducing the gentlemen of the town, who were especially appealed to, and the members themselves, to do all in their power to further the establishment of such institutions.[73]

In July of the next year the ninth annual meeting of the library was addressed by Holland, Knight and Favell upon the same theme, and in September a preliminary public meeting for the promotion of a Mechanics' Institute was addressed by these three together with two of their colleagues, Corden Thompson and Henry Harwood. All five men were physicians.

By October the medical men had obviously attracted great notice, for in that month 163 individuals signed their names to a petition calling for a grand public meeting to debate the question.[74] Once again, a cross-section of the town had responded. Of the 154 known occupations, 28 were medical men, 36 large merchant-manufacturers (14 of whom were substantially concerned in the heavy trades), 29 small manufacturers verging on the 'mester', 9 artisans, 20 small tradesmen (e.g.

from brewer, through auctioneer to victualler), 8 miscellaneous service occupations (e.g. auditors), 11 somehow engaged in law, and 13 who were either teachers or clergymen. Of the first nine names listed, five were the physicians above whose social profiles have already been indicated, and the others were composed of John Read, Samuel Shore, Thomas Rawson and Luke Palfreyman, all four of whom were dissenters and radicals as well as being previously associated with the medical community.[75] Of the 44 initial members of the Sheffield Political Union for Parliamentary Reform in January 1831, 15 put their names to this list of twenty-one months later.[76]

The medical men at once dominated the running of the institution. The first prospectus was drawn up by Thomas Ellis, surgeon, and the first President and regular chairman was George Holland. Of the first six courses of lectures before members, five were by medical men. Most committees, but especially those requiring scientific skills, were run by medical men.[77] Political and religious discussions were excluded from the format of the association, and this would at first appear to contradict the background so far noted. However, when we consider the real need felt to appeal to the whole community for funds and support such exclusions become more understandable. Certainly, the medical men were foremost in the attempt to justify the institute in terms of a general moral rejuvenation in furtherance of utilitarian goals, rather than as part of a reformist or radical programme.[78] At this point, in order for action to remain effective, their explicit statements were no longer in accord with the social image which they had themselves projected. There is little doubt that this process repeated itself in other contexts and via other associations.

Thus, the social profiles of medical men, resulting from their very real need (through time) to establish an identity in a rapidly changing social and economic milieu, were projected outwards into a wide field of local interests and activities, ranging from purely local associations such as the Physical Club, through to pressure groups with national aims, such as the Political Union or the Anti-Corn-Law League. By the 1840s there is no doubt that the medical men had vastly reduced their social marginality. The social need which at first promoted a distinctiveness, produced also, through its very success in concrete areas of social action, status and security. The medical man had attained, using Stacey's phrase, a degree of 'social comfort'. In 1841, at which time he was regarded as one of the most prominent men in Sheffield, Arnold Knight was knighted by Queen Victoria, upon which the *Sheffield Independent* declared: 'The instances indeed are very rare in the ordinary walks of life of men who have done so much for the public as Sir Arnold Knight has done, and his labours have been augmented in value by the manly and consistent character which he has uniformly maintained.' In July 1845 Corden Thompson felt quite able to refuse the Presidency of the Provincial Medical and Surgical Association, at which it was immediately offered to Charles Favell, who, upon accepting the office, gave a lengthy speech on the history of Sheffield and its 'worthies', in which medical men figured largely.[79]

IV

The social profile of the medical men in Sheffield was by no means unique. Even in an area such as Derby, where the economic structure was such as to allow for more non-industrial activity and thus not promote such a definite reaction to a perceived social norm, the medical men were developing a distinct and positive image. As an indication for the period 1790-1830 we may select sixteen men of Derby who were leaders in both medical and scientific pursuits and of whom something is known as to their religious or political affiliations.[80]

Table 3. Profile of the Medical Elite in Derby

Name	Occupation[81]	Religion	Politics[82]
Bennet, W.	Surgeon	Established Church	1812 Reformer
Bent, T.	Physician	Dissenter	1820s-30s Radical
Crompton, P.	Physician	Unitarian	1790s Radical
Darwin, E.	Physician	Deist	1790s Radical
Eaton, T.	Surgeon		1812 Reformer
Fearn, S.W.	Surgeon	Dissenter	1820s Reformer
Forester, R.F.	Physician	Unitarian	1809-30s Radical
Fox, A.	Surgeon		1830s Reformer
Fox, D.	Surgeon	Dissenter	1830s Reformer
Fox, F.	Physician	Established Church	1820-30s Radical
Fox, F.	Surgeon		1790s Radical
Godwin, R.B.	Surgeon		1830s Radical
Hancock, J.	Surgeon	Unitarian	1790s Radical
Hancock, W.	Surgeon	Dissenter	1812 Reformer
Harwood, T.	Surgeon		1830s Radical
Pybus, R.	Apothecary	Unitarian	1812 Reformer

But in the more overtly industrial areas, it would appear, from what has gone before, that the medical men, as a tiny minority, fulfilled a series of social functions going well beyond 'gentlemanly pursuits', certainly functions that can not be easily dismissed by the historian of this period. The design of sections II and III was to show the progress of the medical community through occupational activities, together with the projection of a very definite social image through social action in various fields. The latter served to make more explicit the social identity of the medical man, an identity otherwise placed in jeopardy by his occupational and, invariably, geographical position within the local community.

At this point we might return to the idea of professionalisation as discussed in Section I where the point was made at some length that medicine did not conform to a full definition of the term 'profession' in this period. The social comfort provided through the processes and institutions of a profession was not yet fully obtainable. Greenwood has pointed out that:

> Every profession strives to persuade the community to sanction its authority within certain spheres by conferring upon the profession a series of powers and privileges. . . professional colleagues must support each other vis-a-vis clientele and community. The professional must refrain from acts which jeopardise the authority of colleagues and must sustain those whose authority is threatened.[83]

As a professional culture develops in a particular social context, service and educational groupings emerge within it, until it finally encourages and encompasses those 'organisations which emerge as an expression of the growing consciousness of-a-kind on the part of the profession's members, and which promote so-called group interests and aims'.[84] The present paper has argued that in a situation where the profession is yet forming, these groupings, which also fulfil an identity establishing function for more generally marginal men, may emerge more informally and more widely, encouraging an outgoing approach to community life. Two sets of complex social pressures converge to ensure a positive social role for the provincial medical man.

An important result of this may have been the effect on the class structure which emerged by mid-century. Donald Read is one recent writer in a very long line who have pointed to the 'social union' characteristic of both Birmingham and Sheffield in the period and how this was due to the fact that:

> The metal trades of Birmingham and Sheffield were based (at least until the later years of the nineteenth century) upon a network of small workshops. . .there were many journeymen who could reasonably aspire one day to become small manufacturers themselves. The economic and social structure of Birmingham and Sheffield was thus a unity. . .85

In fact, the relative ease with which the journeyman might become a small producer could promote social disunion. This was especially so at times of demand depression, when confrontation between producers was quite as stark, and had a similar impact, as that which occurred between employer and employee in the more classic situation. Thomas Ward, Sheffield merchant, remarked that, during the bad times of 1820, 'a peculiar depression is added by the workmen making goods and selling them at ruinous prices. . . Trade is at a very low ebb – the paper-knife trade almost at a stand – except among the journeymen who are ruining their masters without serving themselves.'86 Perhaps, then, conflict was resolved, at least partially, through the bridging effect produced via the activities and complex alliances of the medical men, an effect which was itself a function of Sheffield's economic structure.

T.H. Marshall has pointed out that, 'There can be no doubt that, in Mid-Victorian England, the professions were prosperous and respected . . .'.87 But what might be of most importance to the historian is that the *process* whereby the medical men achieved this respect encompassed so much more than medicine. By the mid-century the twin rewards of respect and prosperity had bred the twin characteristics of complacency and rigidity in large sections of the society, including the medical, and a new era had set in.

Appendix – The Medical Community and the Voluntary Associations

Below are listed the total of voluntary associations involved in the estimate in Section III. In one or two cases a description of activities is given where this is not clear, as also is some idea of the formative importance of the medics. In all cases the figure in brackets represents the number of the 43 men meaningfully involved in that association, and the associations are listed according to that involvement. Non-association influences are thus excluded, e.g. 15 of the men were involved in the promotion of itinerant science lecturers in the area, 5 themselves gave courses of public lectures – R Deakin's (surgeon) 40 public lectures on botany.

Literary and Philosophical Society 1822-50 (22) (note that this is where critiques of medical conditions were aired in the 1820s onwards); Mechanics' Institute 1832-50 (18); Sheffield Book Society 1800-50 (15); School of Anatomy and Medicine (12); Physical Club 1830s (10), a very influential grouping of industrialists, teachers and medical men, overwhelmingly scientific and formed in that famous 'middle-class decade'; Society for the Promotion of Useful Knowledge 1804-6 (10), mostly a science forum, see text and notes 41 and 51; Friends of Parliamentary Reform 1809-12 (9), a very important association incorporating a wide variety of occupations in a definite radical stance and facing up to an explicit opposition, the latter, incidently, led by a lawyer; Society for Bettering the Condition of the Poor 1820s-40s (9); Phrenological Society 1820s-40s (9), under which heading 3 more or less formal associations have been subsumed; Medical Institution 1820s-40s (9); West Riding Geological and Polytechnical Society 1830s-40s (7), very much a technical-orientated society in which doctors mixed with coal-mine owners and engineers, and with industrialists in a context wider than Sheffield alone; Cobbett's Club 1810s (6), overtly radical discussions and dinner-parties, five of these six being on the list of 20 in the text; Political Union 1830-2 (6), see text; Mechanics' Library 1823-50 (6); Monthly Club 1790s-1820s (5), a social outlet cutting across many occupations; Shakespeare Club 1820s (5), particularly for the promoters of 'theatrical amusements' generally, and several times in explicit opposition to members of the Established Church; Physiological Society 1830s-40s (5); Lancasterian Schools Movement 1800-20s (4); Humane Society 1810s (4); Anti Slavery Movement 1830s-40s (2); Anti-Corn-Law League 1840s (3); Friends of Civil and Religious Liberty 1820s (2); Church of England Instruction Society 1830s-50 (5), the last two associations showing that Unitarians were quite willing to associate with Anglicans; Peripatetic Society 1840s (2); Sheffield Mechanics' Scientific Society 1820s (2); Society for Literary Conversation (2); People's College 1840s (1).

Notes

1. Arnold Thackray, 'Natural knowledge in cultural context: the Manchester model', *American Historical Review, 79,* 1974, 672-709.
2. R.E. Park, 'Human migration and the marginal man', *American Journal of Sociology, 33,* 1927-8, 881-93.
3. E.V. Stonequist, *The Marginal Man,* New York, 1937, p. xvi *passim.*
4. Modifications since Park have not attempted this level of application, nor have they extended or clearly specified the conception for detailed empirical usage. See E.V. Stonequist, 'The problem of the marginal man',

American Journal of Sociology, 41, 1935, 1-12; M.I. Goldberg, 'A qualification of the marginal man theory', *American Sociological Review, 6,* 1941, 52-8; A.W. Green. 'A re-examination of the marginal man concept', *Social Forces, 26,* 1947-8, 167-71; D.I. Golorensky, 'The marginal man concept, an analysis and critique', *Social Forces, 30,* 1951-2, 333-9; and W.I. Wardell, 'A marginal professional role', *Social Forces, 30,* 1951-2, 339-48. Similar to the approach in this paper, extending the analysis to multiple group and status memberships within a society, is E.C. Hughes, 'Social change and status protest', *Phylon, 10,* 1949, 59-65.

5. E. Greenwood, 'Attributes of a Profession', *Social Work, 2,* 1957, 44-55. In Greenwood's opinion, medicine is today the closest to his conception of the 'ideal profession'. For a summary of the debate over the concept of profession see, J. Ben-David, 'Professions in the class structure of present-day societies', *Current Sociology, 12,* 1963-4, 247-98. Parsons sees the authority relationship between members and client as the crucial index of professionalism because the need to maintain a delicate relationship is the ultimate functional basis of the typical professional attitudes of ethical conduct and disinterested service. On this see Talcott Parsons, 'The Professions and Social Structure' in his *Essays in Sociological Theory,* Glencoe, Illo., 1958. The economic function of the profession tends to be neglected by such authors despite the fact that the guild-like organisations invariably regulate every aspect of the professional's market and work situation. The conferring of status through the prestige attached to the occupation once professionalised serves not only to legitimise the member's authority but also his economic reward.
6. For what is still a good, succinct account of medical institutions in England in this period see A. Chaplin, *Medicine in England during the Reign of George III,* London, 1919, especially pp.8-35. See also Myron F. Brightfield, 'The medical profession in Victorian England as depicted in the novels of the period (1840-1870)', *Bulletin of the History of Medicine, 35,* 1961, 238-56.
7. Sir Zachary Cope, 'How the Society of Apothecaries moulded medical practice in England', in *The Worshipful Society of Apothecaries of London, and the Evolution of the Family Doctor,* London, *c,* 1960, pp. 3-9. The Apothecaries Act of 1815 established an apprenticeship of five years leading to the LSA, and encouraged the development of both London medical schools which would offer anatomical and other facilities, and the provincial medical schools..
8. Chaplin, *op. cit.,* pp. 24-33. As a result of the judgement passed by the Committee of 1834, a Licentiate could be admitted to the examination for the Fellowship without first becoming an MD of either Oxford or Cambridge.
9. S.W.F. Holloway, 'Medical education in England, 1830-1858: a sociological analysis', *History, 49,* 1964, 314.
10. *Ibid.,* 317-19. A vivid impression of the changing social function and position of the provincial medical man is obtainable from the novels of the nineteenth century. Amongst others these would include, Jane Austen's *Emma, Persuasions* and *Pride and Prejudice*; Charles Dickens' *Martin Chuzzlewit*; Elizabeth Gaskell's *Wives and Daughters*; and William Thackeray's *The History of Pendennis,* which tells of how a surgeon develops from the status of a retail druggist. The modern novelist Winston Graham has particularly captured an accurate picture in his five post-war novels on Cornwall in the period 1783-95 entitled *Ross Poldark, Demelza, Jeremy Poldark, Warleggan* and *The Black Moon.* Throughout the volumes, the

young surgeon, Enys MRCS, is constantly involved with establishing a social position in the local context, this resulting in a diversification of his medical activities. On the other hand, Choake, the physician, depends on a series of sinecures. Both prescribe and administer medicines.

11. Cope, *op. cit.*, p. 6.
12. F.N.L. Poynter, 'Medical education in England since 1600', in C.D. O'Malley (ed.), *The History of Medical Education; An International Symposium*, Berkeley, 1970, p. 135.
13. Holloway (*op. cit.*, 324), claims that by the 1830s the private medical schools were no longer able to compete with the hospitals, and that by 1858 'medical education was almost as completely organised within (the hospitals) as it is today' (323).
14. One of the results was that some of the most significant advances in scientific and technical knowledge were increasingly made by trained medical men, many of whom retained their medical practice. The Whitehaven physician William Brownrigg (1711-1800), MD, FRS, carried out important industrial-chemical experiments into coal-mine gases. Peter Shaw (1694-1763), MD,FRS, received his medical degree from Cambridge in 1751, and was an important early chemical lecturer and writer on industrial chemistry – activities which did not prevent him from carrying on a successful practice or becoming physician to George II. Many scientific societes in the provinces, especially those at Liverpool, Manchester and York, were dominated by medical men.
15. For example, *London Evening Post* 21 September 1736, 3, and 21 October 1736. 4. The following paragraph is based on a survey of the *London Evening Post* for the 1730s and 40s, and only those lecturers hitherto overlooked have been noted in the text. Medical and scientific lectures given at institutions have been excluded, e.g. H. Pemberton's at Gresham College on chemistry aimed at 'the Use of Chemistry in the several Trades, whose Works depend upon the Principles of this Art'.
16. *London Evening Post*, 1736-40.
17. Subjects included anatomy, surgery, neurology, physiology, and were not always addressed specifically to medical students.
18. *London Evening Post*, 1737-41. Both Lewis and Alcock are examples of medical teachers and practitioners who were also renowned in other fields. Lewis had strong technological interests and published papers on platina, gold and dye-stuffs, won the Copley Medal in 1754 and was a foremost member of the Society of Arts. See F.W. Gibbs, 'William Lewis, MB, FRS (1708-1781)', *Annals of Science, 8*, 1952, 122-51, and N. Swin, 'William Lewis (1708-1781), as a chemist', *Chymia, 8*, 1962, 63-88. Alcock went to Oxford in 1738 to lecture on chemistry and anatomy, but intermittently lectured in London until at least 1740, advertising his Oxford lectures in the London papers. (His son Thomas, who published his father's memoirs in 1780, was a popular medical lecturer in London in the 1790s.) Alcock was made FRS in 1745 and FRCP in 1754. See N.A. Hans, *New Trends in Education in the Eighteenth Century*, London, 1951, pp. 48-9.
19. The following paragraph is the result of a survey of the *Observer* (London) from 1791 to 1820.
20. Pearson's first advertisements appear in 1800 when he was Physician to St George's Hospital and included medical theory, chemistry, physic and clinical practice. Pearson was a son of John Pearson who had taught William Blair (see text) as an apprentice. George was born in Rotherham, Yorkshire, educated at Doncaster Grammar School and studied under

Cullen and Black at Edinburgh where he received his MD degree in 1773. Elected FRS in 1791, he was a fine chemist and an early supporter of Lavoisier, e.g. in 1794 he published his translation of the *Nomenclature Chimique.* See John Guest, *Historic Notices of Rotherham,* Worksop, 1879, which draws its material from the privately held MS of Pearson's nephew, Henry Bower of Doncaster.

21. *Observer,* 19 and 26 September 1802, 16 January 1803, and 30 December 1804.
22. *Ibid.*, 6 October 1799.
23. *Ibid.*, 1799-1807. Hardie claimed to be a surgeon, a man-midwife and a professional lecturer. At times one hundred or more subscribers were obtained, and the lecturer's design was to establish a regular College of Science.
24. The existence and activities of these institutions have been established from a survey of the *Observer, The Times* (London) and the advertisements in *Annals of Philosophy* prior to 1830. Medical men were predominant, e.g. George Shaw, John Millington and Frederick Accum were foremost in the Surrey Institution. Millington lectured also at the Royal Institution and Guy's Hospital. The independent medical lecturers supported such activities; Henry Clutterbuck (MD, MRCS) continued to give courses at his house in Blackfriars on physic and chemistry until the 1820s.
25. The Physical Society was formed in 1771 and continued in strength until the 1820s. Its scientific and medical discussion and lectures attracted many eminent men, including Astley Cooper, Jenner, Allen (who lectured on Chemistry at Guy's), Marcet and Curry. For an account of its history see J.M.H. Campbell, 'The history of the Physical Society', *Guy's Hospital Gazette, 39,* 1925, 107-19.
26. *Dictionary of National Biography (DNB)*; *Annals of Philosophy,* 10, 1817, 227-8; *Sheffield Iris,* 6 September 1825 and 12 September 1826. Phillips had a strong interest in industrial chemistry and in 1835 brought out a patent for the manufacture of sulphate of soda.
27. *DNB*; *Annals of Philosophy, 6,* 1815, 304; C.H. Spiers, 'William Thomas Brande, leather expert', *Annals of Science, 25,* 1969, 179-203. Brande long continued an interest in medical subjects, being behind the proposal for a Society for the Promotion of Animal Chemistry, admitted a member of the Chemistry to that body.
28. Chaplin, *op. cit.*, pp. 22-3 and 32-5.
29. The economic and social history of Sheffield before 1850 has been sadly neglected. The following provide useful information: Sidney Pollard, *A History of Labour in Sheffield,* Liverpool, 1959, and his *Three Centuries of Sheffield Steel,* Sheffield, 1954; J.C. Hall, *The Trades of Sheffield,* London and Sheffield, 1865; R.E. Leader, *Sheffield in the Eighteenth Century,* Sheffield, 1901; G.I.H. Lloyd, *The Cutlery Trades,* London, 1913; J.H. Stainton, *The Making of Sheffield,* Sheffield, 1924; E.R. Wickham, *Church and People in an Industrial City,* London, 1957; *(White's) Directory of Sheffield for 1837*; E. Goodwin, 'Natural History of Sheffield', *Gentleman's Magazine, 34,* 1764, 157-61 and Sir Arthur Helps, *The Claims of Labour,* 2nd edn., London, 1845.
30. This is based on a survey of the parish by the Church Burgesses in 1736, where the town's population is given as 9,695 and the six parishes as 14,105, producing roughly £100,000 worth of manufactured goods per annum.
31. The first steam engine was introduced by Proctor in 1786, and by the mid-

1830s there existed twenty separate steam grinding wheels together with small ones attached to manufactures, totalling approximately 800 h.p. At this time grinding still employed forty water wheels. The directory of 1837 shows four steam engine manufacturers in the town.

32. Immigration was specially of London silver platers from the 1740s and later of Derbyshire unskilled workers as the lead mining employment decreased. The former group appears to have been of continued importance to at least the early 1790s. From 1800 to the mid-1830s 'great numbers of families from different parts of the country have settled in the town, and embarked on its trade and manufactures'. For the continuation of substantial immigration in later years see A.K. Cairncross, 'Internal migration in Victorian England', *Manchester School, 17,* 1949, 86. The main enclosures were in 1782, 1791, and 1811, and continued into the 1830s.
33. *Census of Population* (1831), *Enumeration Abstract, 2*; G.C. Holland, *The Vital Statistics of Sheffield* (1843), pp. 28-35; Pollard (1959), *op. cit.*, pp. 3-9, and Wickham, *op. cit.*, pp. 19-21. It is difficult to separate the professional from other non-industrial occupations, and this is, anyhow, not necessary when our prime concern is with an occupational group undergoing professionalisation and, on the whole, belonging to the small service group outside of the dominant industrial economy.
34. A contention of this paper is that this non-industrial group was of more importance than historians have noted, not only in such obvious areas as York, Bath, Liverpool, Wakefield, Nottingham and Derby, but also in the more heavily industrialised areas of Sheffield, Newcastle, etc., where the suggested alliance could develop. In many provincial centres it may well have been this group that was formative in the mid-Victorian institutional and authority structure, and thus behind much of the class formation that took place.
35. The major sources for such profiles are brief newspaper notices, and the ones reproduced above are fairly representative. See also John Austen, *Historical Notices of Old Sheffield Druggists,* Sheffield, 1961, and his 'Old physicians and old physic', *Transactions of the Hunter's Archaeological Society, 4,* 1942-6, 189; W.S. Porter, *Sheffield Literary and Philosophical Society 1822-1922,* Sheffield, 1922, and his *The Medical School of Sheffield, 1828-1928,* Sheffield, 1928, and S. Snell, *The History of the Medical Societies of Sheffield,* Sheffield, 1890.
36. As with most of the biographical material in this paper, Holland's life and activities are reconstructed from newspaper references, subscription lists and such like. But see also W. Odom, *Hallamshire Worthies,* Sheffield, 1926, pp. 121-33.
37. As a youth Holland at one time considered a Unitarian college and ministerial training and throughout the 1830s was a strong supporter of Upper Chapel, the main Unitarian chapel in the district. He was an early member of the Sheffield Political Union which promoted the course of radical parliamentary reform. See *Sheffield Mercury* for January, July and November 1831.
38. *Sheffield Mercury,* 5 May 1832. Testimonials from Bouvier, Fouquier and Orfila were included as well as those from well-known Scottish and English physicians such as William Mackenzie, Edward Milligan, John Macintosh and George Longstaff. In addition, thirty-one members of the Hunterian and Physical Societies signed letters in his support, eleven of whom were either Presidents or late Presidents of those societies. The aspects of professionalisation alluded to above are well illustrated in this grouping of men

in support of one of their number, and in their very frequent use of such words as 'profession', 'distinction', 'responsible', 'ethical', 'medical science' and 'scientific medical men'.

39. *Sheffield Register,* 18 May 1792, 3. Of the thirty-three, two were physicians, two were lawyers, and one was William Wilberforce MP. The remainder all appeared to have been merchants or manufacturers such as Samuel Shore, John Booth and John Marshall (iron manufacturers and merchants), John Hoyland, William Law, Thomas Dronfield (silver manufacturers and refiners) and Thomas Holy (industrial chemist). Large subscriptions also came from Liverpool, Hull, York and Bristol.
40. Porter (1928), *op. cit.,* and Snell, *op. cit.*
41. *Sheffield Iris,* 7 April 1803, 2. Similar broad support was obtained at the founding of the Eye Dispensary in 1828 and the Dispensary in 1832. All the Sheffield public medical institutions appear to have been successful in terms of numbers of patients treated, e.g. between 1794 and 1834 67,000 admittances were recorded for the Infirmary.
42. *Sheffield Advertiser,* 11 March 1791. Popular medical lectures had an early history similar and related to those in science, but unlike the latter retained their audiences throughout the nineteenth century, in spite of localised opposition from the medical profession. In Sheffield in the 1790s the medical community strongly opposed the activities of James Graham and Gustavus Katterfelto, although these men were polular enough in other areas – see *Iris,* 5 and 12 August 1796. The 1840s and 1850s witnessed the mushrooming of the activities of itinerant phrenologists, medical botanists, mesmerists, animal magnetists, galvanists and experimental physiologists, all of which, again, calls into question the conception of 'profession' as applied to medicine.
43. *Iris,* 26 May 1807, and 2, 9 and 30 June 1807; T.A. Ward, 'M.S. Notes and Diaries 1800-1869, in 69 volumes', *Sheffield Local Archives (SLA),* S.L.P.S. p. 122 ff., vol. 8, 1807.
44. 'M.S. Minute Book of the Sheffield Society for the Promotion of Useful Knowledge', (*SLA* S.L.P.S. 216/820.6.S.); Joseph Hunter, 'My Contemporaries', Sheffield, 1846 (*Sheffield University Library* MS. 942. 741.H.); *Local Notes and Queries,* 1876, vol. 3, pp. 17-19. Of the thirty-three members, ten were medical men, including David Davis. For further information see note 48.
45. Joseph Hunter, 'M.S. Diary' (*SLA*), February 1806.
46. *Iris,* 21 November 1809, and 28 January, and 3 and 17 July 1810. Two of the strongest supporters were William Newbould, coal and iron merchant, and Charles Younge, one of the largest manufacturers of silver and plated goods.
47. The annual reports of this society were reproduced in the *Mercury* each July in the period 1820-6. For the grinders' asthma and the manner in which such a health problem could serve to bring medicine and industry into contact, see below.
48. Corden Thompson, *An Introductory Lecture on the Studies, Duties and Qualifications of the Medical Practitioner. . . delivered at. . . Sheffield School of Anatomy and Medicine* Sheffield, 1834, p. 4. See also Corden Thompson, *An Address delivered in Mr. Overend's Museum at the Openint of the Sheffield School of Anatomy and Medicine,* Sheffield, 1828; C.F. Favell, *Introductory Address delivered at the Medical Institution, Surrey Street* Sheffield, 1835; Odom, *op. cit.,* pp. 128-9 and 133-4; *(White's) Directory,* pp. 18-4; and *Iris,* 19 February 1828.
49. *Sheffield Independent,* 18 October 1828, 22 August 1829 and 31 October

1829; *Mercury*, 22 September 1832; Ward Diaries, 18 November to 23 December 1828, 25 January to 1 March 1830 and 8 November 1830. Apart from his cutlery manufactory, Barker was closely involved with the Sheffield Lead Works and owned a chemical works at Rugeley.

50. W.J. Bishop, 'Medical book societies in England in the eighteenth and nineteenth centuries', *Bulletin of the Medical Library Association 45*, 1957, 337-50, and *Sheffield Times*, 31 August 1850, 5. The later and detailed history of the workings of such medical associations can be found in Snell, *op. cit.*, and does not concern us here.
51. Minute Book S.P.U.K., (*SLA*), March 1804. According to Joseph Hunter this society 'comprehended nearly all those people in Sheffield who had any literary or scientific turn of mind'. In fact, it linked the medical men with local merchants, tradesmen, cutlers, teachers and lawyers. See Hunter (1846), *op. cit.*, pp. 38-56. For the particular interest of the medical men in local science see below.
52. Ward Diaries, 8 March 1809, 19 September 1826, 8 March 1830, 1 January 1843 and *passim*.
53. *Mercury*, 13 May 1837, *passim*. Occupations have been checked with the directory of that year.
54. *(White's) Directory*, pp. 6-7. Of course, medical men had for some time linked health hazards and industrial processes, e.g. Sutcliffe's paper before the S.P.U.K. of November 1804 on white lead manufacture which intended to find: 'The process for its preparation most economical and least dangerous to the health of the operator. . . without the necessary exposure of the lungs or any part of the surface of the body to the action of the metal' by dissolving in nitrous acid and precipitating in carbonate of potash. In the following year, Dr David Davis gave a more general and critical paper before the same society, entitled 'Sheffield – its situation, manufactures, and their influence on the health and longevity of its inhabitants'. But it was in the 1820s that the medical attitude became more positive and united.
55. 'M.S. Letters T.A. Ward to Joseph Hunter, 1807-1835', (*SLA* S.L.P.S./52), 29 September 1816. John and Charles Fox were major fork manufacturers at New Church Street.
56. *Iris*, 17 September 1822; *(White's) Directory*, p. 8. The most technically successful was that of John Elliott, but by the later 1830s this had yet not been brought into general use.
57. *Mercury*, 5 October 1833.
58. *Annual Reports of the Sheffield Literary and Philosophical Society*, (henceforth *Reports SLPS*), 1838, p. 7; *Mercury*, 7 December 1838, and G.C. Holland, *An Enquiry into the Moral, Social and Intellectual Condition of the Industrial Classes of Sheffield*, Sheffield, 1839.
59. *Reports SLPS*, 1839, p. 6, and 1843, p. 6; *Iris*, 10 August 1841; *Minutes of Council, Sheffield S.L.P.S.*, 1822-72 (*SLA* M.S./S.L.P./195), 4 November 1842, and G.C. Holland, *Mortality of Grinders*, Sheffield, 1842 and (1843) *op. cit.*
60. Of course, there is no suggestion here that the criticisms of the 1830s and 1840s were limited to conditions of industrial employment, and these have simply been given as examples. For instance, in both 1832 and 1849 medical men at once contributed to and criticised the lack of cholera prevention measures instigated locally. In 1846 a separate Health Committee emerged from the Town Council. There were thirty-three members of the Committee, ten of whom were medical men and one other of whom, James Haywood, was a chemist and a regular lecturer on medical subjects.

Of the ten, five were councillors. This committee was behind the publication of James Haywood and William Lee's *A Report on the Sanitary Conditions of the Borough of Sheffield,* Sheffield, 1848. The Report was very critical of sanitary provisions and singled out in its text malfactors, many of them industrialists, by name. In 1849 only 76 cases of death through the cholera epidemic occurred, against 400 in 1832, and this was undoubtedly the result of improved cleansing and increased consultation with medical men.

61. 'Leading' has been defined fairly carefully here as those men of the 120, who appear to have contributed most to both medical and social activities in the town, and who were also important in either political or religious movements. The forty-three persons thus singled out were further divided into those who we knew most about, and those where evidence was more scanty or dubious. The former of those two are the 'leaders' of the table.
62. That is, 'distinctive' not only in terms of the nation but of Sheffield society itself. In terms of total population the number of Unitarians was, of course, very small and in Sheffield there was only one place, Upper Chapel, for Unitarian worship; the census figures of 1851 record total accommodation in Sheffield for the established church as 19,562, for Quakers as 800, for all Wesleyans as 10,479, for Roman Catholics as 950, and for Unitarians as 900. This alone suggests that a figure of eleven out of eighteen known religious affiliations is of some real significance. Also, although Sheffield was and is known for its radical tendencies, these should be qualified; for instance, in both 1792-3 and 1810-12, the opposition to the radical element was strong and in both periods led by established local figures. The almost automatic connection between the Unitarians and the Radicals in the early period was, of course, a result of the political treatment of the dissenters – as Wadsworth has recognised, 'perhaps no group of people was more thorough and, at the same time, discerning and responsible in its support of the cause of liberty than the growing body of dissenters' (K.W. Wadsworth, *Yorkshire United Independent College* London, 1954, p. 61).
63. *The Trial of Redhead Yorke, for a Conspiracy etc. . . before the Hon. Justice Rooke, July 10 1795, York Assizes,* published by the Defendant from Mr Ramsay's Short-Hand Notes, York, 1795, pp. 52 and 164-5.
64. *Iris,* 23 January 1810 and 5 and 26 June 1810. The opposition to reform was led by Robert Brightmore, a lawyer, and included no medical men.
65. *Mercury* 15 January 1831.
66. This column is obviously impressionistic, and political affiliations have been characterised rather than completely represented, although it should be pointed out that *no contradictions* have been discovered. The political movements or institutions considered by the simple labels were as follows: Friends of Revolution (1780s), Friends of Reform (1809-12), Friends of Civil and Religious Liberty (1820s), Political Union (1830-1832), Abolitionist Movement (1832-1833), and Anti-Corn-Law League (1830-1840). In all seventeen of the cases the man involved was either an instigator or committee member of the organisation.
67. *Intended Dinner to H. Brougham (1826) of Friends of Civil and Religious Liberty* (*SLA* M.D./1211/28, Handbills). Barker was from a family of Quakers, but himself an adamant Unitarian, and married the daughter of the surgeon Hall Overend. Luke Palfreyman was of a line of Unitarians and political radicals, his father being imprisoned in 1796 for radical activity, and a foremost member of the Political Union and the Anti-Corn-Law League. Samuel Shore was a very early Unitarian, educated at Norton

Academy and a particular friend of Joseph Priestley who inscribed to him his *History of the Unitarian Church.* Unlike these men, Joseph Read was an Independent and member of a family long engaged in radical causes, including those of the 1790s. See R.E. Wilson, *Two Hundred Precious Metal Years,* London, 1960, pp. 62-5

68. Margaret Stacey, *Tradition and Change: A Study of Banbury,* London, 1960, p. 77. At a later stage she goes on to illustrate and conclude that: '. . .two main factors decide what association a man joins: his political-religious adherence and his social status. Of these social status is dominant, since two men of common adherence will join different associations if their occupational status falls on different sides of the frontier. . .' (p. 89). The fact that the opposite was the case in Sheffield at this time, i.e. that the strength of interest in an activity or movement was easily sufficient to cut across very fundamental occupational divisions, highlights the importance of the social role of the medical community. For a study of the continuing changes in the life of the people of Banbury, see Margaret Stacey, Eric Batstone, Colin Bell and Anne Murcott, *Power, Persistence and Change: A Second Study of Banbury,* London, 1975.
69. J.F.C. Harrison, *The Early Victorians 1832-1851,* London, 1973, p. 131.
70. This includes the twenty men in Table 2.
71. This concept of voluntary associations has here been taken to signify associations having a means whereby affairs of the group are ordered, where membership is voluntary and requires no especial qualification apart from any determined by members, and where there is some continuity; cf. Stacey, *op. cit.,* p. 75.
72. *Sheffield Directories,* 1825 and 1837; *Reports S.L.P.S.,* 1825, and *Annual Report of Sheffield Mechanics' Institute,* 1833. The present paper has neglected a full description of the very important part played by the medical community in the vigorous development of scientific interests; for this see Ian Inkster, 'The development of a scientific community in Sheffield 1790-1850: A network of interests and institutions', *Transactions of the Hunter's Archaelogical Society, 10,* 1973, 99-131.
73. *Mercury,* 9 July, 5 November and 10 December 1831; 7 July and 22 September 1832; *Iris,* 3 July 1832, and *Annual Reports of the Sheffield Mechanics' Library, 2,* 1825.
74. *Mercury,* 13 October 1832.
75. See Table 2.
76. *Mercury* 15 January 1831. On perhaps too little evidence, Betty Tickett has argued a direct causal connection between radical motives and the founding of the Mechanics' Institute, listing five medical men as amongst those connecting the two. On the other hand she includes John Parker MA, JP, as a 'radical'. See Betty Thickett, 'Radical activity in Sheffield 1830-1848', BA dissertation, University of Durham, 1952, pp. 87-9.
77. 'Minute Book of the Sheffield Mechanics' Institute', *I,* 1832-6, (*SLA,* M.D. /231/1), 29 August 1832, and 29 October 1832.
78. For a good example of such spurious justifications and declarations, see Charles Favell, *The Value and Importance of Mechanics' Institutes, An Address before the. . . Sheffield Mechanics' Institute,* Sheffield, 1836. Stacey, *op. cit.,* makes the same point regarding voluntary associations in contemporary English society:'. . . given a common occupational status two men may well join the same association despite differences of religion or politics, provided there are adequate taboos on religious and political discussion' (pp. 89-90). Given that there *was no* such common occupational status in this case, the taboos might be expected to be that much

stronger, especially when the association is being led by an increasingly distinctive socio-religious group. At Sheffield this did not always work. Ironically enough, when the Rev. R.S. Bayley, Congregationalist, gave his lectures to the institute on the Reformation and indulgences, his implications were such that the Roman Catholic Arnold Knight, physician, felt compelled to resign from the committee. However, in the next year, Knight secured the presidency (74 votes) against the competition of Dr Holland (62 votes) and Dr Favell (50 votes). It would appear that a fairly delicate balancing act was being performed (Minute Book, *2* ,1836-45, Committee Meetings, 25 April 1837, 5 November 1838). In fact, most of the medical men in the institute were committed to educational reform, e.g. Holland's energetic promotion of the Worksop, Halifax, Chesterfield, Ackworth and Wentworth Mechanics' Institutes, Favell's founding and support of the Rotherham Institute, and Knight's promotion of plans for national education leading him into a long controversy with the Rev. Thomas Best. More genuine statements can be found in Holland (1843), *op. cit.*, especially pp. 139, 144-6 and p. 244.

79. Odom, *op. cit.*, pp. 125-6, and *Iris,* 31 July 1844. The increasingly established position of the medical community in the 1840s and 1850s, meant that any members who retained in full their earlier radical social profiles, found themselves in a potentially deviant social position. This would appear to be true of G.C. Holland after about 1843-4.
80. The sixteen were selected from a larger group of forty-one men, all leading medical men and all engaged in local scientific activities. Reliable political and religious material could be included for only sixteen of these. The local scientific activities surveyed in this period were as follows: The Literary and Philosophical Society (1787-1830), the New Literary and Philosophical Society (1808-30), the Mechanics' Institute (1825-30), support given to itinerant lectures in science (1825-35), Natural History Society (1825-40), Chesterfield Literary and Philosophical Society (1830-5), Chesterfield Mechanics' Institute (1830-5), and were of the involved type stipulated above for Sheffield.
81. Darwin, Crompton and Bent were of fairly established families, although Darwin was new to Derby society. Some were engaged in more than one occupation; Crompton had banking interests, Forester was for a time in partnership as an ironmaster, Francis Fox the physician was also a manufacturing chemist and closely involved, commercially, with the introduction of gas lighting, as well as a patentee of various devices, and Richard Pybus was also a manufacturing chemist, druggist and patentee. These industrial connections might have served to reduce occupational marginality as medical men identified with industrial change.
82. Labels have only been applied when an individual was foremost in one at least of the following: Committee of Protestant Dissenters (1790), Corresponding Society/Society for Political Information (1791-2), Friends of Reform (1809-10), Petition for Peace/Peace Movement (1812), Spanish Subscription (1823), Anti-Corn-Law Movement (1825-7) and Abolitionist Movement (1830).
83. Greenwood, *op. cit.*
84. *Ibid.*, 51. Greenwood goes on to include informal groupings as a component of the profession where 'membership in these cliques is based on a variety of affinities. . . (including). . . family, religious or ethnic background; and personality attractions'; cf. text and footnotes 48,59,77-9, and appendix.
85. Donald Read, *The English Provinces 1760-1960, A Study of Influence,*

London, 1964, p. 35. See also Pollard (1959), *op. cit.*, and Lloyd, *op. cit.*
86. 'Ward-Hunter Letters' (*SLA*). 29 March 1818, and 26 February and 11 July 1820.
87. T.H. Marshall 'The Recent History of Professionalism in Relation to Social Structure and Social Policy', in his *Sociology at the Crossroads*, London, 1963, p. 153.

6 GENERAL PRACTITIONERS AND CONSULTANTS IN EARLY NINETEENTH-CENTURY ENGLAND: THE SOCIOLOGY OF AN INTRA-PROFESSIONAL CONFLICT

Ivan Waddington

It is curious that the development of the general practitioner in the late eighteenth and early nineteenth centuries – arguably the most important development within the medical profession during this period – has been so little studied by medical historians. In part, this failure to analyse the development of the general practitioner in a systematic way probably derives from the reluctance of medical historians to abandon the traditional tripartite classification of physicians, surgeons and apothecaries as a framework for the study of the medical profession in this period, for such a classificatory scheme necessarily makes it difficult to come to grips with many of the problems posed by the development of a new type of practitioner who was neither physician, nor surgeon, nor apothecary. In this paper it will be suggested, following Holloway's argument,[1] that the tripartite classification is not very useful for an understanding of the changing structure of the medical profession in the first half of the nineteenth century, and that the profession may be more adequately analysed in terms of the emergence of a new professional structure, based on the differentiation between general practitioners and consultants. Following this, the main body of the paper will then be concerned with a systematic analysis of the social, economic and political situations of these two groups, and of the relationship between them which, it is hoped, will throw some light on other aspects of the development of the profession, and in particular on the interrelated problems of intra-professional conflict and the development of the medical reform movement, both of which figure prominently in the history of the profession in the first half of the nineteenth century.

It is not difficult, of course, to see why medical historians have almost always used the tripartite classification as a framework for the analysis of the medical profession in the period prior to 1858. Thus it is true that during this period the law recognised only three types of medical practitioners: physicians, surgeons and apothecaries. It is equally true that this tripartite structure was institutionalised in the structure of the three major controlling bodies engaged in granting qualifications to practice medicine and surgery, namely the Royal College of Physicians, the Royal College of Surgeons and the Society of

Apothecaries. Nevertheless, as Holloway has argued, to make the assumption that this classification corresponds to what practitioners actually did, rather than simply to their formal, or legal status, is extremely misleading.

As noted above, the three legally recognised types of practitioner in England were physicians, surgeons and apothecaries. These three groups were organised in a hierarchical structure, with physicians forming the 'first class of medical practitioner in rank and legal pre-eminence'.[2] By the early nineteenth century, the practice of the physician was held to be 'properly confined to the prescribing of medicines to be compounded by the apothecary, and in superintending operations performed by surgeons in order to prescribe what was necessary to the general health of the patient, or to counteract any internal disease'.[3] Physicians were traditionally held to be scholars and gentlemen; Dr Newman says they 'used their heads not their hands', and that they 'advised rather than did'.[4]

It is, however, doubtful whether many physicians limited their practice to advising and prescribing. In 1834, John Sims, physician to St Marylebone Infirmary pointed out to the Select Committee of that year that 'there are very few physicians who practise as such' and he added that 'the principal part of the practice is in the hands of the general practitioners'.[5] Thirteen years later Professor Christison held that there were a great number of physicians practising in England as general practitioners; the title of MD, he said, particularly in the provinces, did not exclude the practice of surgery by a member of the College of Physicians.[6] John Burns, Professor of Surgery at Glasgow University, similarly held that in the greater part of England, as in Scotland, physicians 'practise everything that comes to them'.[7] There is good reason to believe that, especially in the provinces, there were many physicians whose practice included surgery and midwifery, as well as pharmacy. In the north of England, in particular, there were numerous physicians holding Scottish degrees who were engaged in general practice.[8] In 1847, James Bird pointed out that 'Ever since the year of 1815, there has been a bone of contention between the Scotch and Irish graduates and the Society of Apothecaries'[9] because the Scottish and Irish graduates in general practice objected to the fact that under the 1815 Apothecaries' Act they were required to pass the examination of the Apothecaries' Society or risk prosecution for illegally practising as apothecaries. Readers of Trollope will recall that Dr Thorne, though a graduated physician, took over the former practice of a 'humble-minded general practitioner' in Greshamsbury, and that the Doctor 'As was then the wont with many country practitioners. . .added the business of a dispensing apothecary to that of physician'.[10] It was not unknown for even medical graduates of Oxford to practise as general practitioners.[11]

Nor was general practice among physicians confined to the provinces, for in London Scottish graduates were in general practice in sizeable numbers from the 1760s onwards.[12] By the 1830s and 1840s, even the most eminent physicians in London were performing the minor operations of surgery[13] and they did 'not scruple to take fees in surgical cases'.[14] In 1834, Neil Arnott, a licentiate of the College of Physicians, was of the opinion that so many physicians were practising generally that 'before long the body called physicians will wear out'.[15]

A similar story emerges if we examine the situation of those practitioners who were legally designated as surgeons. According to the law, the proper sphere of practice of the surgeon was held to consist generally in the cure of all outward diseases, and in the use of surgical instruments in all cases where this was necessary.[16] There is, however, little reason to believe that many surgeons confined their practice to pure surgery. Thus in 1834, Benjamin Brodie pointed out that of surgeons practising in England, 'only a limited number can confine their practice to surgery, even in London; and very few, if any, can do so in the country', and he went on to observe that the activities of the physician and the surgeon had become increasingly intermingled since 1780.[17] Sir Anthony Carlisle held that the most eminent surgeons in London practised not only surgery, but medicine too, and he admitted that he saw as many patients 'in the character of a physician, as of a surgeon'. He held that the 'distinctions between what ought to belong to a physician, and what belong to a surgeon, are quite undefinable'.[18] Fourteen years later, George James Guthrie, a councillor of the Royal College of Surgeons, stated that when called in to consultation, he was not in the habit of ascertaining beforehand whether it was a medical or surgical case. Asked if, when called into a case, he found it to be internal without any external appearances, he would decline to accept it, Guthrie stated 'If I thought I was capable of curing the disease I should attempt it; if I thought I was not, I should desire them to send for some one else.'[19] Honoratus Leigh Thomas, who was on two occasions President of the College of Surgeons, was frequently called into consultation by J.F. Clarke for medical cases. Clarke wrote that Thomas was a poor surgeon, but that he was a 'shrewd practitioner in medical cases to which his practice was mainly limited'.[20]

Perhaps the most eminent of all nineteenth-century surgeons was Sir Astley Cooper, yet not even he limited his practice to surgical cases.

While he was lecturer on surgery at St Thomas's Hospital, Cooper encouraged poor patients to come to him at his home for gratuitous advice; in this way he was able to maintain a supply of interesting cases for the hospital. To induce the poor to come to him, Cooper purchased and continually kept at hand a stock of common medicines, which he bestowed liberally 'on them whose means would not allow them to take his prescriptions to the chemist's shop in the usual way'.[21] There is little reason to believe that James Bird was exaggerating when he suggested that 'it is difficult to define what pure surgery is. The fellows of the College of Surgeons, if they thought proper to practise as pure surgeons, might call themselves pure surgeons if they pleased; but I think very few of them practise it.'[22]

If the most eminent London surgeons rarely confined their practice to pure surgery, this was even less common among rank and file surgeons. In 1834, when there were some six thousand members of the College of Surgeons practising in England and Wales,[23] the President of the College estimated that only two hundred of these confined their practice to surgery; the rest were general practitioners.[24] Fourteen years later, John Ridout, a fellow of the College of Surgeons, agreed that 'by very far the larger proportion' of members of the College were general practitioners.[25] In 1848, James Bird, a member of the council of the National Institute of Medicine, Surgery and Midwifery, provided the Select Committee of that year with a breakdown of its membership; two-thirds of the members of the Institute, which was an association of general practitioners, were members of the College of Surgeons.[26] That many surgeons dispensed their own medicines is indicated by the fact that in his evidence before the same committee, Guthrie stated that when he was President of the College, he offered to make up a register of surgeons who were general practitioners, but was prevented from doing so because it was held that he would 'show them up to the apothecaries to be prosecuted if they had not their license'.[27] This conclusion, as well as the considerable confusion surrounding medical practice at this time, is aptly conveyed by Bird's comment that 'Scotch graduates and Irish graduates, and members of the College of Surgeons who are not also licentiates of the Society of Apothecaries, and licentiates of the Apothecaries' Society who are not members of the College of Surgeons, are all practising indiscriminately, as general practitioners in this country, in medicine, surgery and midwifery'.[28] John Nussey, Master of the Society of Apothecaries, stated in 1834 that it was estimated that as early as 1812-13 there were some 12,000 general practitioners.[29]

There is little doubt that many surgeons acted as general practitioners without the licence of the Apothecaries' Society; nevertheless a considerable number of practitioners obtained the double qualification after the passing of the Apothecaries' Act in 1815. In 1834, some 3,500 members of the College of Surgeons also held the licence of the Society of Apothecaries,[30] while in 1848 James Bird estimated that there were between 14,000 and 15,000 general practitioners in England and Wales, and that 'more than half of the 14,000 possessed the double qualification'.[31]

It is clear that the practice of the great mass of surgeons was indistinguishable from that of the apothecaries. A correspondent of the *Lancet* in 1841 told of a practitioner in Cornwall who had passed the Apothecaries' Hall in 1828, but had never obtained the diploma of the College of Surgeons, 'nor ever attended a surgical lecture, or the surgical practice of an hospital; nor, indeed, ever saw any surgical operation excepting those performed behind the counter of a drug shop – yet he calls himself a "surgeon", has "*SURGEON*" on his street door, and holds the appointment of a medical and surgical attendant on the poor in this district.'[32] The correspondent went on to enquire whether such practice was illegal; the *Lancet* correctly replied that there were no laws to prevent apothecaries or anyone else practising surgery. There is little doubt that the vast majority of apothecaries availed themselves of this opportunity; such examples of general practice on the single qualification could be multiplied at great length.

It is clear that in the first half of the nineteenth century, the traditional divisions within the profession were becoming increasingly irrelevant to what practitioners actually did. This is not to say that the traditional terminology ceased to be used; even the *Lancet,* since its foundation in 1823 a vigorous and consistent campaigner against the unreal separation of medicine and surgery, was forced to use the traditional terminology. But it is to say that in this case, as in many others, changes in terminology lagged behind changes in the structure of the profession, and that the terminology was, therefore, misleading. If the terms 'physician', 'surgeon' and 'apothecary' remained common in the medical literature of the nineteenth century, it was becoming increasingly difficult to find more than a handful of 'pure' practitioners in any branch.

What was happening during this period, as Holloway has pointed out,[33] was that as the traditional tripartite structure was steadily breaking down, so it was being replaced by the modern professional structure, based on the differentiation between general practitioners and consultants. In large part, the changes within the structure of the profession appear to have been brought about by the changing pattern of demand for medical care, which in turn was associated with the changes in the class structure brought about by the Industrial Revolution. Thus in the early nineteenth century there was a widening of the demand for medical care, largely because of the development of a sizeable middle class. Early in the nineteenth century, Robert Masters Kerrison commented on the 'augmentation of the middle orders of the community', and pointed to the importance of this development for medical men. One effect of the growth of the middle classes was, he said,

> a proportionate increase of sickness, amongst people, who were unable to procure medical aid, by feeing Physicians as often as their situation required professional care, and the Members of the Royal College of Physicians, having made no diminution in their accustomed fee, to meet the actual wants of persons in this class of society, they were compelled to resort to others for advice.[34]

There thus existed a large and growing number of people who required qualified medical care, but who were unable to engage pure physicians and surgeons on the terms traditionally charged. The middle class demand was essentially for medical men able and willing to engage in all branches of practice, and to charge for their services at modest rates. Miss Franklin has correctly noted that the 'expansion of the industrial community. . .produced a greater demand less for the highly qualified physician than for the family doctor',[35] a position which came to be filled by the general practitioner.

Moreover, it was, of course, also in the self-interest of those practitioners who attended the middle classes to practise generally. Pure physicians and surgeons had traditionally treated small numbers of wealthy clients and had charged high fees. Those practitioners who attended middle-class families, and perhaps occasionally the families of more highly paid manual workers, had of necessity to charge fees which were very much lower. As we shall see later on, many general practitioners in the early nineteenth century earned only very modest incomes and it is doubtful whether many surgeons could afford to turn away medical cases, or whether apothecaries could afford to turn away the minor cases of surgery. As the *Lancet* pointed out in 1842 in reviewing the development of the profession, many surgeons had 'found it desirable, both for their own interest and that of the public, to conjoin the business of the apothecary with their own'.[36]

The result of the changing pattern of demand for medical care was that the great mass of surgeons and apothecaries, as well as a good many physicians, broadened the scope of their practice, and became general practitioners treating large numbers of families and charging modest fees. Other changes, however, were also occurring within the medical profession during this period. Thus the growth of hospitals in the eighteenth and nineteenth centuries had given rise to a much smaller, but very important, class of consulting physicians and surgeons who, as McKeown has pointed out, owed their position as consultants primarily to their hospital appointments.[37] Thus in the late eighteenth and early nineteenth centuries the traditional tripartite professional structure was steadily being eroded and replaced by the modern professional structure, based on the differentiation between the general practitioner and the hospital-based consultant. Having thus outlined in general terms the changing structure of the profession, we must now go on to examine in some detail the situation of consultants and general practitioners in the first half of the nineteenth century.

Whichever aspect of their situation we examine, we find that consultants enjoyed considerable advantages over their colleagues in general practice. Generally, the consultants figured on the staffs of the charitable hospitals of London and the main provincial cities, and since the advantages which they enjoyed derived, in large part, from their positions within the hospitals, it is necessary to examine the network of relationships which centred on these situations.

The early charitable foundations had for centuries employed physicians and surgeons and remunerated them in cash and kind for their attendance. However, in the newer hospitals, the doctors were generally unpaid. Moreover, the older foundations failed to revise their salary rates to take account of the current value of the services they were receiving, and though small payments continued to be made in some hospitals, physicians and surgeons gradually acquired honorary status.[38]

The direct rewards for medical attendance were thus at best modest. However, as hospitals developed as centres of medical education in the late eighteenth and early nineteenth centuries,[39] the rewards from teaching came to be very large. In 1844, Dr Carus observed that at St Bartholomew's, 'the physicians are not paid, as is the case so frequently in England, but several young men and surgeons attend their lectures, study their treatment of the patients, and pay them for this privilege a considerable fee, so that in this way a few thousand pounds are easily made in the course of a year.'[40] In the early 1820s, the theatre of St Thomas's Hospital 'was crowded in every part by upwards of four hundred students of the most respectable description',[41] all of whom paid three guineas or more, the greater part of which went to the lecturer.

In addition, surgeons in the larger voluntary hospitals in London often received large fees from apprentices. Paget recalled that in the 1830s the usual fee for the four or five years' pupilage was 500 guineas, and for resident pupils 1,000 guineas.[42] In January 1826, Frederick Tyrrell, a surgeon at St Thomas's Hospital, received £1,050 from or on behalf of William Tice James and in 1830 Tyrrell received the same sum again when he accepted James Dixon as an apprentice. In December 1825 John Alexander Harper's premium to Aston Key, a surgeon at Guy's was £1,000. In 1822, Edward Stanley, surgeon at St Bartholomew's Hospital received £700 on behalf of William Pennington, while William Money received £800 on behalf of Thomas Egerton in the same year. Benjamin Travers accepted Samuel Solly as an apprentice for 500 guineas, but in 1834 Solly himself required 600 guineas as a premium. The regulation fee paid to the leading hospital surgeons in London appears to have been in the order of 500 to 600 guineas; sums in this range were repeatedly paid to Green, Abernethy, Earle and Stanley.[43] In the provinces, fees were lower, but still considerable. When Thomas Ash was apprenticed to Samuel Dickenson, surgeon to the Birmingham General Hospital, in 1815, the premium was £210.[44]

The direct income from teaching could thus be very considerable. Nevertheless, the greater part of the incomes of consultants was derived not from teaching, but from private practice. Here again, a position in one of the larger teaching hospitals was important. In the first place, teaching enabled consultants to establish contacts with large numbers of students, who in later years sent their own wealthy private patients for remunerative consultations. Secondly, the lay governors of the charitable hospitals were both wealthy and influential; holding an appointment at one of these hospitals meant that there was a good chance of becoming medical adviser to the lay members of the board. Thirdly, a hospital appointment was an excellent advertisement in attracting wealthier clients. Abel-Smith has correctly noted that it 'became known by private patients that the hospital staffs possessed the most advanced knowledge. Charitable work became the key to fame and fortune.'[45]

Few consultants confined their work to consulting practice, but also acted as general practitioners to the nobility and wealthy merchants.[46]

In this capacity consultants, whether physicians or surgeons, practised both medicine and surgery, but rarely pharmacy or midwifery. General practice was frequently financially rewarding; as a writer in the *Quarterly Review* pointed out in 1840, consultants were the regular attendants 'among those who have the advantage of ease and affluence'.[47] Consulting practice was also lucrative. In 1813, Sir Astley Cooper performed the operation for stone upon Mr Hyatt, a wealthy merchant, for which he received 1,000 guineas. The two physicians who attended with him each received £300.[48]

The combined income from teaching, consulting, and general practice was often very high. In 1815 Sir Astley Cooper's income exceeded £21,000.[49] Like other consultants, Cooper treated a wealthy rather than numerous clientele; his biographer recalled that it was not unusual for him to receive only five fees in the course of a morning's work, 'and yet the sum he received might be large, for they almost all paid in cheques'.[50] Although Cooper's income in 1815 was quite exceptional, other consultants earned large incomes. On occasions Abernethy earned £10,000 and Liston nearly £7,000 a year.[51] Among the consulting physicians, Matthew Baillie, early in the century, earned £10,000 a year for many successive years,[52] while in the 1820s and 30s, Sir Henry Halford, for many years the President of the Royal College of Physicians, 'made his £10,000 a year regularly'.[53] William Chambers, physician to St George's Hospital and an Elect of the Royal College of Physicians, also had a very lucrative practice in London. Between 1836 and 1851 his income is known to have ranged between seven and nine thousand guineas a year.[54]

Many consultants thus enjoyed market situations which were extremely lucrative. In addition they held a virtual monopoly of the major political offices within the profession. As we shall see below, general practitioners were excluded from the governing councils of the Royal Colleges of Physicians and Surgeons, and the offices which the consultants held within the Colleges enabled them to perpetuate the advantages which they enjoyed, sometimes at the expense of other members of the profession. Thus on 6 December 1822, the Court of Examiners of the College of Surgeons resolved that only those lectures on anatomy which had been delivered in the winter session would be recognised by the College.[55] This made of no avail the courses given by excellent teachers in the private schools during the summer session. At a protest meeting of members of the College held at the Freemasons' Tavern in February 1826, two speakers expressed concern at the effect this regulation was having on Joshua Brookes's famous school in Great

Marlborough Street.[56] Their fears were not unjustified, for as Cope has noted, by this regulation 'the well-known and popular courses of Joshua Brookes were banned and that celebrated teacher was ruined'.[57]

In 1824 the Court of Examiners of the College of Surgeons passed a second regulation which, like that of 1822, had the effect of restricting competition from other teachers, and thus of preserving the very lucrative teaching monopoly of the consultants in the larger hospitals. The regulation stated that in future the only schools of surgery to be recognised by the Court would be those of London, Dublin, Edinburgh, Glasgow and Aberdeen, and that certifictes of attendance at lectures, and certificates of attendance upon the surgical practice of an hospital, would only be received if the teachers and hospitals were in one of the above recognised schools.[58] The *Lancet* wrote of these regulations that 'we never beheld any resolutions more hostile to science, or more decidedly avaricious',[59] and, addressing its words to the Examiners of the College, it pointed out that 'gentlemen, you have been, or are still, hospital surgeons yourselves, and therefore you have passed this measure for your own advantage, and that alone'.[60]

Thus consultants not only found that the economic rewards of the profession were frequently very high, but they also enjoyed a virtual monopoly of the key political offices within the profession. These were, however, not the only benefits accruing to consultants, for in the hospitals they also had access to research facilities which were normally unavailable to general practitioners and which, with the development of modern medicine early in the nineteenth century, came to be of ever-increasing importance.[61]

If we now compare the situation of consultants with that of general practitioners, we find a number of important differences. Unfortunately it is not easy to generalise about the economic situation of the latter group, since the available evidence on incomes of general practitioners is very fragmentary. Nevertheless, two points are clear. The first is that the incomes of general practitioners varied considerably, depending on the type of practice. Thus a small practice in a fashionable seaside or inland spa town would be worth considerably more than a larger practice in a predominantly working-class industrial area. Similarly a rural practice in a sparsely populated area involved considerable work for comparatively small returns. That cathedral, seaside and spa towns offered a better livelihood to medical men is indicated by the fact that throughout the nineteenth century these towns attracted more practitioners, per head of population, than industrial areas or thinly populated rural districts.[62] Medical men tended to go where the returns from practice were greatest.

The second point is that those practitioners with less fashionable practices frequently earned only small incomes. John Pendennis, the father of Thackeray's hero, was a surgeon-apothecary in the west of England and had a 'very humble little shop'. He had 'for some time a hard struggle with poverty; and it was all he could do to keep the shop and its gilt ornaments in decent repair, and his bed-ridden mother in comfort.' It was not until, by accident, he received the patronage of Lady Ribstone, who introduced him into 'the good company of Bath', that he began to prosper.[63] Many practitioners kept open shop in order to supplement their meagre incomes. Thus Pendennis 'not only attended gentlemen in their sick-rooms, and ladies at the most interesting periods of their lives, but would condescend to sell a brown-paper plaster to a farmer's wife across the counter – or to vend toothbrushes, hair powder, and London perfumery.'[64] A correspondent of the *Lancet* in 1840 held that surgeons should be compelled 'to abandon the sale of patent pills, pastilles, perfumery, soap, etc.',[65] a view which was frequently expressed, since retailing was held to be degrading to members of a profession. Since, however, retailing provided an important source of income for many poorer practitioners, it was a practice which could not be given up without serious financial loss.

In 1900 H.N. Hardy recalled that 'in the early part of the century, medical men were content to accept rates of payment which, though known to be inadequate, were often as much as could possibly be spared from too scanty wages'.[66] Many practitioners found their incomes insufficient to enable them to make adequate provision, upon their deaths, for their families. The Society for the Relief of Widows and Orphans of Medical Men, which was formed to provide for the families of deceased practitioners who found themselves in straitened circumstances, reported in the early 1840s that 'one in four of the members of the society has left a widow or orphans claimants on its funds'.[67] Hardy indicates that poverty persisted among many medical men throughout the whole of the nineteenth century. Thus at the end of the century there were three charitable societies in London alone which aimed at 'relieving cases of pecuniary distress among medical men, their widows and orphans'. Hardy commented that as 'the number of those relieved by the London societies alone amounts to between 450 and 500 every year, and as there are always far more applicants even for doles of £5 and £10 a year than can be satisfied out of the funds at the disposal of the various societies, it is evident that in the battle of life but too many practitioners and their families come to grief.'[68]

If the market situation of many general practitioners was not, in economic terms, very rewarding, this was not, however, their main complaint. Though comment on their modest financial situation was not infrequent, the major grievance of general practitioners centred on the relationship between themselves and the medical corporations, and in particular, the Royal Colleges. To understand the causes of these complaints, we have to relate the policies of the Royal Colleges to the changing structure of the profession outlined at the beginning of this paper.

As we have seen, the traditional structure of the medical profession had involved the differentiation of three groups of practitioners, namely physicians, surgeons and apothecaries, and corresponding to this differentiation there were three major controlling bodies – the Royal College of Physicians, the Company of Surgeons (from 1800 the Royal College of Surgeons), and the Society of Apothecaries – each of which had its own charter or Act of Parliament and its own by-laws, and each of which granted licences to practise in the particular branch for which it was responsible. Moreover, not only were physicians, surgeons and apothecaries organised in quite separate medical corporations, but the policies of the medical corporations had long been designed to maintain the barriers separating the different types of practitioner and the different branches of practice. Thus throughout the eighteenth century, no apothecary could secure the licence of the Surgeons' Company without ceasing to be a member of the Society of Apothecaries.[69] Similarly, no apothecary or surgeon could take out a licence from the College of Physicians without relinquishing his membership of the Apothecaries' Society or the Company of Surgeons. In 1756 William Hunter had to pay forty guineas to withdraw from the Company of Surgeons because he wished to practise as a physician,[70] while in 1795 the College of Physicians approved the refusal of the President, Sir George Baker, to examine an apothecary who applied for a licence to practise physic, and instructed the officers of the College to prepare a statute authorising the like rejection of any person employed as an apothecary or surgeon.[71] In the early nineteenth century, George Mann Burrows and Charles Locock were among Surgeons and/or the Society of Apothecaries prior to becoming licentiates of the College of Physicians.[72] In 1834, the College of Physicians had still not modified this regulation.[73]

Throughout the first half of the nineteenth century, both Royal

Colleges persisted in this traditional policy of trying to maintain the separation of medicine and surgery, and in particular, of rigidly separating both these branches of practice from what were regarded as purely manual or trading activities. To further this policy of maintaining the purity of physic and surgery, the Royal Colleges of Physicians and Surgeons excluded from their governing councils those who practised as apothecaries, and those who practised midwifery. In the College of Physicians, this had traditionally been effected by restricting the fellowship of the College to graduates of Oxford and Cambridge, that is, to gentlemen by whom the manual work involved in midwifery and pharmacy was seen as degrading. In 1771, however, the by-laws of the College were revised, and the ban on the practice of midwifery and pharmacy was made explicit. The by-laws stated that no person practising midwifery was to be admitted to the fellowship, that physicians practising as apothecaries were not to be admitted, and that fellows who entered on practice as apothecaries were to be expelled.[74]

In the Company of Surgeons, it had been stipulated by a by-law of April 1748, that 'no person practising as an apothecary or following any other trade or occupation besides the profession or business of a surgeon, shall be capable of being chosen into the Court of Assistants (Council)'.[75] On its foundation in 1800, the Royal College of Surgeons retained the emphasis on pure surgery and, indeed, retained the by-law of 1748.[76] In his evidence before the 1847 Select Committee, John Ridout stated that the College of Surgeons had persistently shown itself unwilling to undertake an efficient examination with regard to general practitioners as well as surgeons: '. . .it was proposed in 1812, 1813 and 1814, that they should then undertake the superintendence of the medical as well as the surgical education of the surgeon or surgeon-apothecary; but the opinion of the council at that time was, that they wished to confine their attention to surgery exclusively, and they have continued to express a similar opinion down to the present time'.[77] In his evidence before the same committee, Benjamin Travers, President of the College, held that 'there is perfect eligibility to the fellowship, but not perfect eligibility to the council; a man, for example, must have nothing to do with the practice of pharmacy to take a seat in the council'.[78]

Nor did the Royal Colleges change their attitude towards the practice of midwifery. In the 1820s, after a suggestion that the Royal College of Physicians should examine in midwifery, a committee reported to the College, giving a plethora of historical information, tending to show that 'the object of the College has been to confine the fellows to the pure practice of physic.'[79] In 1834, the attitude of the President, Sir Henry Halford, was equally uncompromising. Thus he said of midwifery that

> I think it is considered rather as a manual operation and that we should be very sorry to throw anything like a discredit upon the men who have been educated at the Universities, who have taken time to acquire their improvement of their minds in literary and scientific acquirements, by mixing it up with this manual labour. I think it would rather disparage the highest grade of the profession, to let them engage in that particular branch, which is a manual operation very much.[80]

The College of Surgeons also maintained its opposition to the practice of midwifery. Thus Guthrie concluded his observations on surgeons who practised midwifery with the comment that 'with all possible respect for this class of gentleman, I must say, that I should be exceedingly sorry to see the first accoucheur in this town president'.[81] The attitude of the College towards surgeons who practised as apothecaries and accoucheurs – that is surgeons in general practice – was, perhaps, most clearly pointed out in a long statement issued by the Council of the College on 26 April 1826. The statement was a reply to a demand by members of the College that officers of the College should be elected annually by the whole membership. The Council held that the

> . . .evident object of this representation is the subversion of the present government of the College, and the substitution of election to offices of control and responsibility, by members, who for the most part exercise the professions of apothecaries and accoucheurs. There can be little doubt, that in the event of such an innovation, the Institution would soon cease to be a College of Surgeons or of Surgery.[82]

In the College of Surgeons, the official reason for the exclusion from the Council of those who practised midwifery and pharmacy, was that such practitioners had no time or means to devote to specialising in the study of surgery.[83] There is little doubt that the emphasis on pure surgery had, in fact, been instrumental in achieving one of the objects in terms of which it was justified, namely, raising the status of surgery, for in this process, the differentiation of the role of the surgeon from that of the tradesman had been of major importance. Thus at the beginning of the eighteenth century, the status of surgery was very much lower than that of medicine, the surgeons being still associated with the barbers in the Company of Barber-Surgeons. Just over a century later the status of surgery had risen so considerably that Paget was able to recall that when he entered St Bartholomew's in 1834, 'the main interest and power of the Hospital were surgical. . .the teaching and importance of medicine were made to seem very inferior to those of anatomy and surgery; and the contrast was sustained in many things outside the Hospital'.84

In the College of Physicians, the problem had been not so much to raise the status of physicians, as to maintain the high status which they had for long enjoyed. The physician traditionally was a learned and cultured gentleman; the ban on midwifery and pharmacy, for those who aspired to the rank of fellow, was aimed at preserving this status by obliging fellows to abstain from those tasks which were considered manual.

Thus throughout the first half of the nineteenth century, both Royal Colleges persisted in their traditional policies of trying to maintain the pruity of their respective branches of practice.This point is of major importance, for what the Royal Colleges were, in effect, trying to do, was to maintain the traditional structure of the profession, based on the distinctions between physicians, surgeons, and apothecaries, at the very time that changes in the wider social structure were effecting changes in the structure of the profession itself. As we have already seen, in the first half of the nineteenth century, the traditional tripartite structure of the profession was breaking down, and giving rise to a new structure, in which the major groups were generalpractitioners and consultants. Of these two, the general practitioners were by far the larger group, and by the 1830s probably provided some 90 per cent of the qualified medical care in England. But the role of the general practitioner necessarily involved not only medicine and surgery, but also, in a period in which the birth rate had not yet declined, a good deal of midwifery, and generally pharmacy too. Thus the development of the general practitioner was a process which necessarily undermined the tripartite structure, since the development of general practice involved a breaking down of the rigid barriers separating the different branches of practice. The Royal Colleges, dominated by the consultants, bitterly resisted this development, however, for they feared that the incorporation of manual and trading elements into the doctor's role threatened the high status which physicians had long enjoyed, and which surgeons had recently attained. Thus the attempt on the part of the Royal Colleges to maintain the traditional tripartite structure was simultaneously an attempt to stem the rise of the general practitioner, a policy which, not surprisingly, not only gave rise to a good deal of resentment among a large section of the profession, but also gave birth to a very long and very bitter campaign for medical reform on the part of the general practitioners.

The effect of the policies of the Royal Colleges was, of course, to deny to the great majority of the profession any direct control over the decision-making processes within the two most influential medical corporations; general practitioners were thus effectively divorced from the exercise of power within the profession. While the consulting surgeons, who held a qualification in surgery only, were eligible for election to the Council of the College of Surgeons, the general practitioner, who often held, in addition to his surgical diploma, a qualification in medicine from the Society of Apothecaries, was excluded. Commenting on this situation, the *Lancet* maintained that the Royal Colleges

> . . .have discovered the most extraordinary ground for creating professional distinction that ever entered into the mind of man. With them the chief qualification for eminence in the healing art is ignorance of one or the other half of it. A physician need not know much of physic; an entire ignorance of surgery will be sufficient to give him a respectable standing; a surgeon need not possess any real knowledge of surgery, but if he be sufficiently ignorant of physic – if he do not know the gout from the measles – that will render him 'pure', and make him eligible to receive the highest appointments; but a 'general practitioner' – a man who is so preposterous as to understand both physic and surgery – is fit only to become a 'subordinate'.[85]

In addition to the Royal Colleges, there was, of course, the Society of Apothecaries. Few general practitioners, however, looked to the Society to represent their interests, for not only that the Society retained a constitution more typical of a city trading company than a medical corporation, but it also had a long association with the apothecary as the inferior member of the medical profession, and as recently as 1815 had been a party to the Apothecaries' Act, which defined more clearly than ever the inferior status of the apothecary.[86] In 1848 James Bird explained that many general practitioners preferred that title to the more traditional one of 'surgeon-apothecary', since the term 'apothecary' 'was intended to denote an inferior grade'.[87] The long association with 'Rhubarb Hall', as the *Lancet* called it, was more a hindrance than a help to the general practitioner in his attempts at professional advancement.

In the first half of the nineteenth century there was thus no medical corporation to represent the interests of the general practitioners. As James Bird observed, 'neither the College of Surgeons nor the College of Physicians has any sympathy with the general practitioners; the interests of that body have at all times been placed in abeyance, and for want of a recognised position they have hitherto been disregarded in all communications with the Government.' He added that '. . .whenever any medical question, or any question affecting the public health, is brought before the Legislature, there is no body, no head, to represent the interests of nine-tenths of the profession'.[88] The situation of general practitioners within the medical profession was clearly pointed out by the *Lancet* when it asked 'where have the surgeons in general practice their head-quarters? What body presides over their interests? Alas! they have no local habitation, and no presiding body. Positively, the only set of men who have a right to be considered as forming the medical profession in this country have neither representatives nor protection.'[89]

In addition to excluding the general practitioners from their Councils, both Royal Colleges persistently refused to make provision for the type of education required for general practice. Thus the general practitioner required an education and examination in medicine, surgery, midwifery, and pharmacy, but no medical corporation required, or would examine on, an integrated course embracing all these subjects. As we saw previously, the College of Surgeons consistently refused to make provision for the medical as well as the surgical education of the general practitioner, preferring to confine its interest to pure surgery, while the College of Physicians maintained its traditional policy of examining in physic only. Thus the general practitioner was compelled to go to the Apothecaries' Society for his examination in medicine and pharmacy, and to the College of Surgeons for a separate examination in surgery. Moreover, for the first quarter of the nineteenth century, neither the Royal Colleges nor the Society of Apothecaries would have anything to do with the practice of midwifery. In 1827 the Apothecaries' Society required evidence from candidates for their diploma that they had received training in midwifery, but the Royal Colleges maintained their traditional examinations in physic and surgery only.

Educationally, as well as politically and socially, the general practitioner was rejected.

Given this situation, it is hardly surprising that consultants and general practitioners should view the tripartite institutional structure of the profession in radically divergent ways. Although, as we have seen, the nineteenth-century consultant no longer corresponded to the traditional 'pure' physician or surgeon, there were, nevertheless, a number of similarities between the consultants and the pure physicians and surgeons which meant that consultants, unlike general practitioners, could be assimilated into the traditional professional structure without any great difficulty. Thus consultants normally held a qualification in either medicine or surgery, but rarely both; they could thus continue to designate themselves as physicians or surgeons, to enjoy the legal privileges of those groups and, indeed, to maintain the fiction that medicine and surgery were separate branches of practice which were best left to separate groups of practitioners. Moreover, like the pure physician and surgeon, consultants rarely practised pharmacy or midwifery; hence they were not excluded from the Councils of the Royal Colleges and, indeed, as we have seen, the consultants held a virtual monopoly of positions on these Councils throughout the first half of the nineteenth century. Moreover, if the consultants could be easily assimilated into the traditional institutional structure of the profession, there was also no reason why they should desire to change it. Not only did the hierarchical tripartite structure legally confirm their superior status over the general practitioners, but it continued to reward them economically, socially and politically, as well as it had rewarded the pure physician and surgeon. In short, a radical change in the institutional structure of the profession offered little hope to the consultants of improving their situation, while there was every possibility that such a change might involve a radical change in the balance of power within the profession, and that general practitioners might benefit at the expense of the consultants.

The situation of general practitioners was quite different. As we have seen, general practitioners were a new group, who had developed in the late eighteenth and early nineteenth centuries, alongside a much older professional structure. The general practitioner was not a physician, nor a surgeon, nor an apothecary. Nor even was his situation within the medical profession adequately conveyed by the term surgeon-apothecary, in spite of the fact that by the middle of the nineteenth century most general practitioners held a qualification from both the College of Surgeons and the Society of Apothecaries. For the title of surgeon-apothecary implies that the role of the general practitioner could be defined in terms of the traditional categories within the profession; this, however, is quite wrong, for in combining the roles of surgeon and apothecary, a completely new type of practitioner had emerged. As a contemporary observer put it, general practitioners were 'a new class. . .different from any hitherto known, formed by a combination of the three already in existence, but having no exact resemblance to any of them'.90

For this reason, it is suggested that the term general practitioner was more accurate than that of surgeon-apothecary; the new terminology reflected the emergence of a new role, and one that could not be fitted into the traditional professional structure. Thus while there was a place in the traditional structure for the surgeon and for the apothecary, there was no place for the practitioner who combined both roles. A correspondent of the *Lancet,* writing on behalf of the general practitioners, summed the situation up in the following manner. General practitioners, he said,

> . . .form the principle body of medical practitioners, and yet, strange to say, we are the outcasts of every medical corporation. The College of Physicians spurn us; no merit, however exalted, could ever qualify one of our body for admission to the sanctum sanctorum of Pall Mall East. The College of Surgeons, although it accepts our guineas, and permits us to be called 'Members', excludes us from ever having a voice in its proceedings. Even the Worshipful Company of Apothecaries turn up their noses at us. But is this as it ought to be? Assuredly not; and it only remains for ourselves, calmly and deliberately, but firmly and in unison, to bring the matter forward, and the system must be altered.91

Thus in the first half of the nineteenth century, the structure of the medical profession involved a basic contradiction. On the one hand, the institutional framework of the profession corresponded to the traditional professional structure, which involved a rigid separation of the roles of the physician, the surgeon and the apothecary. On the other hand, however, these traditional divisions were, in practice, rapidly breaking down as a new professional structure emerged in response to changes in the wider network of relationships in which practitioners were involved. Hence the contradiction between a new professional structure and traditional professional institutions organised on quite different principles. It was this structural tension within the profession which gave rise to the medical reform movement among general practitioners, for since the general practitioner corresponded to none of the three traditional types of practitioner, there was no place for him within the traditional institutional structure. Unwanted by all the medical corporations, the general practitioner was at best tolerated, never welcomed as a full member of the professional community.

Thus from the last three or four decades of the eighteenth century,92 the general practitioners began a long struggle for medical reform aimed at achieving recognition of what they held to be their rightful place within the profession. Among other things, they put forward demands for the democratic reform of the medical corporations, for the reform of medical education and licensing, and for the abolition of the traditional tripartite structure based on the differentiation between physicians, surgeons and apothecaries. This latter point is of major importance, for since the general practitioner could not be fitted into any of these traditional categories, it was only by breaking down these traditional divisions, and replacing them with ones which corresponded more closely to the new professional structure, that general practitioners could hope to achieve recognition of general practice as a legitimate and honourable medical activity.

Inevitably, one consequence of this reform movement within the profession was the polarisation of general practitioners and consultants into opposite camps, for as we have seen, the consultants had a strong vested interest in maintaining the established institutional structure of the profession. Moreover, the fact that the consultants monopolised the key political offices within the Royal Colleges enabled them to effectively resist, for many years, the general practitioners' demands for reform. The result was that the struggle for medical reform was, as is well known, very lengthy, frequently very bitter and even, on occasions violent. It is hoped that the foregoing analysis of relationships between general practitioners and consultants helps to make clear the social structural basis of this struggle which, perhaps more than anything else, dominates the history of the medical profession in the first half of the nineteenth century. A more detailed analysis of the development of the medical reform movement, and of the general practitioners' eventual success with the passage of the 1858 Medical Act is, however, beyond the scope of this paper.

One or two more general theoretical points can, however, be made at this stage. The first is that the conflicts which arose within the medical profession were by no means unique to medicine, for the changing pattern of demand for professional services in the nineteenth century produced some similar changes, resulting in similar tensions, within other professional groups. Perhaps most striking are the similarities in the development of the legal and medical professions, for like medicine, the legal profession was a very old profession with a traditional institutional structure. As Carr-Saunders and Wilson have pointed out, the development of these professions

> . . .was anything but smooth. . . On reflection it appears that what happened in both cases was the early segregation of practitioners, advocates, and physicians, whose function at a later date was realised to be specialist. But the association of these specialists, having attained great power and prestige, attempted to inhibit the development of general practitioners of law and medicine of whose services the public had need. When they could not prevent their appearance, they tried to keep them subservient and the history of both professions is largely concerned with the problems so brought about.[93]

It would seem likely that similar problems may frequently arise when new professional groups emerge alongside established professional structures.

Finally, it is necessary to emphasise that the conflict between consultants and general practitioners within the medical profession can be understood only by analysing the structure of the profession itself; it cannot be understood by reference to the personalities of any particular individuals involved in the conflict. Though elementary, this point continues to require emphasis, since many medical historians, in describing the development of the medical reform movement among general practitioners, have deemed it necessary to document in some detail the personal virtues and vices of one or two particular individuals, which, either explicitly or implicitly, are used as explanatory variables.[94] The resort to individual characteristics in order to 'explain' social phenomena, is, however, a resort of theoretical bankruptcy. As Norbert Elias has pointed out, 'specific maladjustments, discrepancies of one kind or the other between professional institutions and the needs they serve, and tensions between groups of people engendered by those discrepancies, impose their pattern upon individuals. They, not individuals as such, are the main levers of a profession's development.'[95] It is only by analysing the socially structured tensions within a profession that we can understand why and how the institutional framework emerged and changed from period to period. If we do this, we come 'face to face. . .with people struggling, often in vain, to adjust their inherited institutional framework with all its incongruities to what they feel to be their own needs'.96 It is hoped that this paper, by analysing the structure of relationships between general practitioners and consultants, help us to understand more adequately the social basis of the struggle for reform within the medical profession in the first half of the nineteenth century.

Notes

1. S.W.F. Holloway, 'Medical education in England, 1830-1858: A sociological analysis', *History, 49,* 1964, 299-324.
2. J.W. Wilcock, *The Laws Relating to the Medical Profession,* London, 1830, p. 30.
3. *Ibid.*, pp. 30-1.
4. Charles Newman, *The Evolution of Medical Education in the Nineteenth Century,* London, 1957, p. 1.
5. *Select Committee on Medical Education,* 1834 (602-I), part I, Q.2257.
6. *Third Report from the Select Committee on Medical Registration and Medical Law Amendment,* 1847-8 (702), Q. 1969, 1975.
7. *Ibid.*, Q. 2269-75.
8. See Holloway, *op. cit.*, 307-8.
9. *First and Second Reports from the Select Committee on Medical Registration and Medical Law Amendment,* 1847-8 (210), Q. 1215.
10. Anthony Trollope, *Doctor Thorne,* London (Everyman's Library edition), 1967, pp. 25-6.
11. *Association Medical Journal, 4,* (new series), 1856, 253.
12. See Ivan Waddington, 'The struggle to reform the Royal College of Physicians, 1767-1771: A sociological analysis', *Medical History, 17,* 1973, 107-26.
13. *Third Report from the Select Committee,* Q. 1977.
14. *Select Committee on Medical Education,* 1834 (602-II), part II, Q. 5980.
15. *Ibid.* (602-I), part I, Q. 2470.
16. This is a very general outline of a rather complex legal situation. For a more detailed examination of the legal status of the surgeon, see Willcock, *op. cit.*, pp. 56-8.
17. *Select Committee on Medical Education,* 1834 (602-II), part II, Q. 5679-83.
18. *Ibid.*, Q. 5980-1.
19. *First and Second Reports from the Select Committee,* Q. 268-9.
20. J.F. Clarke, *Autobiographical Recollections of the Medical Profession,* London, 1874, p. 113.
21. Bransby Blake Cooper, *The Life of Sir Astley Cooper,* London, 1843, vol. I, p. 235.
22. *First and Second Reports from the Select Committee,* Q. 1227.
23. For details of membership of the College, see the *Select Committee on Medical Education,* 1834 (602-II), part II, Appendix 44, p. 87.
24. *Ibid.*, Q. 4791, 5372.
25. *First and Second Reports,* Q. 495.
26. Of a total membership of 1,350, there were 866 members who were also

members of the Royal College of Surgeons. See the *First and Second Reports*, Q. 1124.
27. *Ibid.*, Q. 136.
28. *Ibid.*, Q. 934.
29. *Select Committee on Medical Education*, 1834 (602-III), part III, Q. 11-12.
30. *Ibid.* (602-II), part II, Appendix 44, p. 87.
31. *First and Second Reports*, Q. 1061-4.
32. *Lancet*, 1841-2, *i*, 422.
33. Holloway, *op. cit.*, 313-4.
34. Robert Masters Kerrison, *Observations and Reflections on the Bill. . .*, London, 1815, quoted in B. Hamilton, 'The medical professions in the eighteenth century', *Economic History Review*, *4*, (new series), 1951, 141-69.
35. Rachel E. Franklin, *Medical Education and the Rise of the General Practitioner*, PhD thesis, University of Birmingham, 1950, p. 4.
36. *Lancet*, 1842-3, *ii*, 720.
37. T. McKeown, ' A sociological approach to the history of medicine', *Medical History*, *14*, 1970, 342-51.
38. B. Abel-Smith, *The Hospitals 1800-1948*, London, 1964, p. 6.
39. Although Guy's Hospital officially accepted students in 1769, Dr Newman holds that the 'generally accepted date for the beginning of regular medical teaching in a hospital in England is 1772, when Dr George Fordyce started courses of lectures on chemistry, materia medica and the practice of physic in St Thomas's.' See Charles Newman, 'The hospital as a teaching centre', in F.N.L. Poynter (ed.), *The Evolution of Hospitals in Britain*, London, 1964, pp. 187-205.
40. Max Neuberger, 'C.G. Carus on the state of medicine in Britain in 1844', in E. Ashworth Underwood (ed.), *Science, Medicine and History, Essays in Honour of Charles Singer*, London, 1953, vol. II, pp. 263-73.
41. Sir Samuel Squire Sprigge, *The Life and Times of Thomas Wakley*, London, 1899, p. 77.
42. Stephen Paget (ed.), *Memoirs and Letters of Sir James Paget*, London, 1901, p. 82
43. *Lancet*, 1917, *i*, 434.
44. Franklin, *op. cit.*, p. 60.
45. Abel-Smith, *op. cit.*, pp. 18-19.
46. The fact that consultants did not confine their practice to consulting work was a source of friction between general practitioners and consultants. See Ivan Waddington, 'The development of medical ethics: A sociological analysis', *Medical History*, *19*, 1975, 36-51.
47. *Quarterly Review*, *67*, 1840-1, pp. 58-9.
48. Cooper, *op. cit.*, vol. II, pp. 158-9.
49. *Ibid.*, p. 193.
50. *Ibid.*, p. 157.
51. J.F. Clarke, *op. cit.*, pp. 115-6.
52. *Munk's Roll*, vol. II, p. 404.
53. Sir George Clark, *A History of the Royal College of Physicians of London*, Oxford, 1966, vol. II, p. 655.
54. *Munk's Roll*, vol. III, p. 197.
55. Zachary Cope, *The History of the Royal College of Surgeons of England*, London, 1959, p. 43.
56. *Lancet*, *9*, 1825-6, 725-43.
57. Cope, *op. cit.*, p. 43. See also Cope's essay: 'The private medical schools of London (1746-1914)', in F.N.L. Poynter (ed.), *The Evolution of Medical*

Education in Britain, London, 1966, pp. 89-111.
58. *Lancet, 2*, 1823-4, 104-6.
59. *Ibid., 2*, 1823-4, 105.
60. *Ibid., 2*, 1823-4, 199.
61. For an analysis of the significance of hospitals as centres of research, see Ivan Waddington, 'The role of the hospital in the development of modern medicine: A sociological analysis', *Sociology, 7*, 1973, 211-24.
62. Walter Rivington, *The Medical Profession*, Dublin, 1879, pp. 3-4. Differences in the provision of medical care ranged from one medical man to 210 persons in Buxton, to one to 6,295 in Aberdare.
63. W.M. Thackeray, *Pendennis*, London, 1906 edn., pp. 6-7.
64. *Ibid.*, p. 6.
65. *Lancet*, 1840-1, *ii*, 107.
66. H.N. Hardy, *The State of the Medical Profession in Great Britain and Ireland in 1900*, Dublin, 1901, p. 70.
67. *Lancet*, 1841-2, *ii*, 100.
68. Hardy, *op. cit.*, p. 15.
69. H.C. Cameron, *Mr. Guy's Hospital, 1726-1948*, London, 1954, p. 83, note 14.
70. Cope, *op.cit.*,
71. Clark, *op. cit.*, vol. II, p. 621
72. *Select Committee on Medical Education*, 1834 (602-I), part I, Q. 4306, and *ibid.* (602-III), part III, Q. 335-7.
73. *Ibid.* (602-II), part II, Q. 4902-6.
74. Clark, *op. cit.*, vol. II. p. 566
75. *First and Second Reports*, Q. 11.
76. *Ibid.*, Q. 11.
77. *Ibid.*, Q. 804
78. *Ibid.*, Q. 1393.
79. Clarke, *op. cit.*, vol. II, p. 664.
80. *Select Committee on Medical Education*, 1834 (602-I, part I, Q. 232.
81. *Ibid.* (602-II), part II, Q. 4801.
82. Sprigge, *op. cit.*, p. 198.
83. *Select Committee on Medical Education*, 1834 (602-II), part II, Q. 4801.
84. Paget, *op. cit.*, p. 62.
85. *Lancet*, 1842-3, *ii*, 719-22.
86. See S.W.F. Holloway, 'The Apothecaries' Act, 1815: a reinterpretation', *Medical History, 10*, 1966, 107-29, and 221-35.
87. *First and Second Reports*, Q. 1248-51.
88. *Ibid.*, Q. 1152.
89. *Lancet*, 1842-3, *i*, 722.
90. *Ibid.*, 1839-40, *ii*, 795-7.
91. *Ibid., 9*, 1825-6, 701.
92. Elsewhere I have suggested that the struggle to reform the Royal College of Physicians in the period 1767-71 may be regarded as one of the earliest attempts by general practitioners to achieve a measure of medical reform. See Ivan Waddington (1973), *op. cit.*, note 12 above.
93. A.M. Carr-Saunders and P.A. Wilson, *The Professions*, Oxford, 1933, p. 304.
94. Thus Dr Newman claims that Thomas Wakley was the 'driving force', behind the medical reform movement. He was, we are told, 'a lifelong agitator', an 'ill-intentioned fellow. . .and a perfect nuisance'. His trouble 'was probably the internal contradictions in his make-up'. (Newman, *op. cit.*, note 4 above, pp. 140-1. Such detailed descriptions may or may not be accurate, but they are for the most part irrelevant to an understanding

of the medical reform movement, and they often have the unfortunate consequence of directing our attention away from the socially structured tensions within the profession.

95. Norbert Elias, 'Studies in the genesis of the naval profession', *British Journal of Sociology*, *1*, 1950, 291-309.
96. *Ibid.*, 293.

INDEX OF PERSONS

GENERAL INDEX